THE ROAD TO MEDICAL STATISTICS

THE WELLCOME SERIES IN THE HISTORY OF MEDICINE

Forthcoming Titles

The Home Office and the Dangerous Trades
By P. W. J. Bartrip

The Regius Chair of Military Surgery
in the University of Edinburgh, 1806-55
By Matthew H. Kaufman

Cultures of Child Health in Britain and
the Netherlands in the Twentieth Century
Edited by Marijke Gijswijt-Hofstra and Hilary Marland

Dental Practice in Europe at the End of the Eighteenth Century
Edited by Christine Hillam

The Wellcome Series in the History of Medicine series editors are
H. J. Cook, C. J. Lawrence and V. Nutton.
Please send all queries regarding the series to Michael Laycock,
The Wellcome Trust Centre for the History of Medicine at UCL,
24 Eversholt Street, London NW1 1AD, UK.

THE ROAD TO MEDICAL STATISTICS

Edited by
Eileen Magnello and Anne Hardy

Amsterdam – New York, NY 2002

First published in 2002
by Editions Rodopi B. V., Amsterdam – New York, NY 2002.

Magnello, Eileen and Hardy, Anne (eds) © 2002.

Design and Typesetting by Michael Laycock,
The Wellcome Trust Centre for the History of Medicine at UCL.
Printed and bound in The Netherlands by Editions Rodopi B. V.,
Amsterdam – New York, NY 2002.

Index by Dr Laurence Errington.

British Library Cataloguing in Publication Data
A catalogue record for this book is available from the British Library
ISBN: 90-420-1597-7 (Paper)
ISBN: 90-420-1208-0 (Bound)

The Road to Medical Statistics –
Amsterdam – New York, NY:
Rodopi. – ill.
(Clio Medica 67/ ISSN 0045-7183;
The Wellcome Series in the History of Medicine)

Front cover image by Michael Laycock.

© Editions Rodopi B. V., Amsterdam – New York, NY 2002
Printed in The Netherlands

All titles in the Clio Medica series (from 1999 onwards) are available to
download from the CatchWord website: http://www.catchword.co.uk

Contents

List of Contributors

Anne Hardy is a Reader in the Wellcome Trust Centre for the History of Medicine at UCL. Her principal interests are in the history of disease and epidemiology, including medical statistics; she is currently working on a history of the salmonellas in Britain.

Edward Higgs is a Lecturer in the Department of History at the University of Essex. His main research interests are the generation of state statistics, including medical statistics, in nineteenth and twentieth century Britain. He is also engaged in a broader study of the surveillance of society by the British State since 1500.

Philip Kreager is a Lecturer in Human Sciences, Somerville College, and Oxford University, currently directing a Wellcome Trust Project on Population Ageing in Indonesia.

Eileen Magnello is a Research Associate of the Wellcome Trust Centre for the History of Medicine at UCL. She has been interested in measurement and statistics for more than two decades, and worked as a statistician before writing her DPhil thesis on Karl Pearson. She has published several papers on Pearson and *A Century of Measurement: An Illustrated History of the National Physical Laboratory* (2000).

J. Rosser Matthews received his PhD in the history of science and medicine from Duke University and is the author of *Quantification and the Quest for Medical Certainty* (1995). During the 2000-2001 academic year, he was a Lecturer in the History of Medicine Department at the University of Wisconsin-Madison. In the summer of 2001, he took up residence at the National Institute of Heath in Bethesda, Maryland as a Stetten Post-Doctoral Fellow in the history of twentieth century medicine. While at the NIH, he examined the history of scientific debates about the relationship between asphyxia and cerebral palsy and its impact on medical malpractice and public policy.

i

John E Senior tutors history of science, medicine and technology in Oxford. He is a Research Associate of the Wellcome Unit for the History of Medicine, and a member of Linacre College, Oxford. His interests in medical statistics arose from his DPhil thesis, *Rationalising Electrotherapy in Neurology, 1860-1920*, and research in evidence-based health care.

Andrea Rusnock teaches in the History Department at the University of Rhode Island. She is the editor of *The Correspondence of James Jurin (1684-1750), Physician and Secretary of the Royal Society* (1996), and she has recently completed a book entitled *Vital Accounts: Measuring Health and Population in Eighteenth-Century England and France.*

Preface

There has been a growing recognition of the importance of mathematical and statistical methods in the history of medicine, particularly in those areas where statistical methods are a *sine qua non* such as epidemiology and randomised clinical trials.[1] Despite this expanding scholarly interest, the development of the mathematical and statistical technologies in the biological sciences has not been examined systematically. The essays in this book are all concerned with the use of these quantitative technologies and focus on medical and clinical cultures from the seventeenth to the twentieth centuries.

The role of statistics in the modern randomised clinical trial has recently received a fair amount of attention. William Coleman discussed the work of the experimental physiologist, Gustav Radicke, who devised some of the earliest statistical tests for therapeutic trials in Germany in 1858.[2] Desirée Cox-Maksimov has shown how Major Greenwood implemented the Pearsonian statistical paradigm in his clinical trials for the Medical Research Council.[3] Harry Marks has examined some of the statistical concepts that influenced the development of the clinical trial in the United States.[4] The use of state medical statistics in the development of civil registration in England and Wales has been examined by Eddy Higgs while Rosser Matthews explored the use of quantitative methods in medicine in the late-nineteenth and early-twentieth centuries.[5] Much of the existing scholarship on other quantitative issues in medicine has tended to focus on the use of probability either for actuarial or philosophical purposes to show, for example, how the notion of chance became a part of medical discourse. Ian Hacking has discussed the use of actuarial methods in eighteenth and nineteenth century Britain for measuring the quantum of sickness[6], and Ted Porter has shown how the work of actuarialists in mid-Victorian Britain became more mathematical[7]. The use of probability in modern biology is discussed by Gerd Gigerenzer, Zeno Swijtink, Theodore Porter, Lorraine Daston, John Beatty and Lorenz Krüger in *The Empire of Chance*[8]. In particular, the use of 'chance' was invoked in controversies concerning vitalism, mechanism, teleology, essentialism and levels of organisation.

Historians have also shown that by the end of the nineteenth century the statistical thinking of biologists and other groups of scientists was shaped by their rejection of determinism and the subsequent acceptance of the philosophical tenets of indeterminism. Hacking argued that at the end of the nineteenth century, statistical patterns emerged and it was then possible to regard the world as not necessarily deterministic. Ted Porter, notably, has also shown how the rise of statistical thinking for such individuals as Adolphe Quetelet led to the rejection of the doctrine of determinism.[9] Apart from these philosophical considerations of probability in medicine or in biology, however, the practice of using various mathematical or statistical technologies in the biological sciences has been given very little consideration.

The use of mathematics in medicine can be traced back to the Hippocratic *Epidemics*. In antiquity, mathematics was used to determine the effects on human bodily health of the motions of the stars and planets. During the Renaissance, Sanctorius pioneered the study of iathromathematics (medical mathematics) which was used for medical meteorology intended to measure the weather, morbidity and mortality as well as the functioning of the human body. Around the same time various graphical techniques were also being developed to record these measurements in tables, graphs and maps. By the eighteenth century, mathematical and quantitative methods were often being applied to medical purposes: the French mathematician and encyclopaedist, Jean Le Rond D'Alembert (1717–1783) calculated the advantages and disadvantages of inoculation by determining the probability of the risks of dying in a month from smallpox or from inoculation. His results indicated that inoculation was a probabilistic advantage in preventing death by smallpox. Apart from such use of probability, however, medical statistics in the modern sense is a more recent development, and should be distinguished from the systematic collection and deployment of vital statistics which first developed as a feature of mid-Victorian preventive medicine. It was only towards the end of the nineteenth century that the discipline of mathematical statistics was developed, to be widely adopted by the medical community in the second half of the twentieth century.

The word 'statistics' is derived from the Italian word *statista* which was first used during the sixteenth century, to designate a Statist, or statesman, who was concerned with describing affairs of the state. The word was co-opted into German shortly afterwards (*Staat*), and the Latin adjective *statisticus* came into fashion in seventeenth century Italy. It was at this time that a closer association between mathematics and medicine began, when the first steps were taken, independently in Germany and England, to assess national welfare and standing – the welfare and standing of the *state* – by means of number. On the one hand this led, in Germany, to the development of political economy, on the other, in England, to the development of vital statistics. Towards the end of the eighteenth century, Gottfried Achenwell, then Professor of Law and Politics at Göttingen, introduced the term *Statistik* as a separate and distinct branch of knowledge to designate 'a mixture of constitutional history, the elements of political economy and statescraft'. 'Statistics' was thus applied to everything that pertained to the state.

The early English usage of numbers in medicine has traditionally been considered to be that of vital statistics, in its nineteenth century sense, which belongs essentially to the history of epidemiology and of preventive medicine. Thus the work of John Graunt and William Petty in the late-seventeenth century follow through that of Gregory King, Thomas Nettleton and James Jurin in the eighteenth century to William Farr at the General Registrar Office between 1839 and 1879. John Graunt's work on the London Bills of Mortality in the seventeenth century has been considered by many later statisticians to be one of the first treatises on vital statistics. In the first essay in this volume, Philip Kreager argues that Graunt's work cannot be described as statistical, and suggests a more complex origin for the English statistical tradition. Graunt used the term 'political arithmetick' to describe his work – a term coined for him by his friend William Petty. Kreager considers his work in its intellectual context, arguing from the textual evidence that Graunt derived his method from seventeenth century mercantile bookkeeping and Francis Bacon's natural history. Although Graunt's work may be described as quantitative, it is not statistical in the sense that the term has been used since the 1830s.

Andrea Rusnock's essay on the early-eighteenth century work of Thomas Nettleton carries further this differentiation of quantitative and statistical methods in the early 'vital statistical' texts. Nettleton's 'Merchant's Logick', reminiscent of Graunt's political arithmetic, introduced a newer kind of quantitative argument into medicine. Following a serious epidemic outbreak of smallpox in England in 1722, educated English society was riven by debates about whether inoculation should be undertaken. Rusnock argues that the mathematical approach indicated by Nettleton's merchant's logic and deployed in subsequent debates on smallpox was a critical step in the development of medical statistics.

Other eighteenth century preoccupations also furthered the development of statistics: games of chance and, more pragmatically, the emergence of an insurance industry, stimulated the growth and application of probability, more especially in France, in the works of Abraham DeMoivre and Pierre Simon LaPlace. At the same time, early English insurance offices and friendly societies were using probability for the construction of life tables – a technique suggested by Graunt and implemented by Edmond Halley. Towards the end of the eighteenth century, the Scottish landowner and first president of the Board of Agriculture, Sir John Sinclair, introduced the words 'statistics' and 'statistical' into the English language with the publication of his 21 volume *Statistical Accounts of Scotland* (1791 to 1798). For Sinclair, statistics was 'an inquiry into the state of a country *for the purpose of ascertaining the quantum of happiness enjoyed by its inhabitants, and the means of future improvement.*'[10]

Competition between France and England, sharpened by the French revolution and the descent of Europe into war after 1793, led English society to consideration of its military manpower and population resources in the last decade of the century. Debates about the size of the British population were fuelled, in part, by the publication of Thomas Robert Malthus's *Essay on the Principle of Population* in 1798. Suggestions for a national census were opposed by those who feared the results would show England's population to be smaller than was commonly believed, thus encouraging her enemies, and by those who thought it would trespass on the liberty of the individual. Nevertheless, Parliament approved a Census Bill in 1800 and the first population census of England and Wales was taken in 1801, inaugurating a national record which was to be of critical importance to the emergence of the modern vital-statistical methodology in the late-1840s.

In the early-nineteenth century continued warfare in Europe, the rapid growth of British industrial cites and population, and the discovery of poverty, deprivation and disease as a price of unregulated urban development and economic progress served to keep a lively interest in numbers and methods of social measurement alive among the ruling classes. In 1829, Francis Bisset Hawkins published his *Elements of Medical Statistics* which, John Eyler suggests, was the first English textbook on vital statistics. Hawkins predicted that the application of statistics to medicine would permit the compilation of accurate histories of disease, as well as the evaluation of the impact of living conditions on life, health and labour, the determination of the effectiveness of treatments, and provision of a basis for reliable diagnoses.[11] Five years later in 1834, Malthus, together with Charles Babbage (who developed the universal calculating machine – a precursor to the computer) and the Belgian statistician, Adolphe Quetelet, founded the Statistical Society of London, which quickly established a notable tradition of statistical enquiry.[12] Among the Society's early concerns was the absence, in Britain, of civil registration procedures for births, marriages and deaths, and it recommended the introduction of a national registration system with a central office in London. Following legislation in 1836, civil registration was introduced, the notification of births, marriages and deaths was required, and the General Register Office was established, giving England and Wales a system of demographic recording unique in Western Europe at that time.

The appointment of William Farr as Compiler of Abstracts to the Registrar General in 1839 was a landmark in the development of English preventive medicine and medical statistics.[13] Although deficiencies in the national system of collecting statistics continued to be remedied for the rest of the century, the demographic material which the new registration system provided permitted assessments of the health and welfare of the people of England and Wales on a scale unimaginable only decades previously. More importantly, the cause of death material allowed detailed analysis of national, regional and local trends and differences, and a pin-pointing of critical problems of disease and public health.

The annual reports of the Registrar General, and the Compiler's 'Letters' to the Registrar General, are, together with the reports the Chief Medical Officer published from 1858, the central texts for the history of public health and disease in Victorian England. In the third essay in this volume, Eddy Higgs argues that the Registrar General's reports were also the central text of Victorian and Edwardian medical statistics, and examines the factors which influenced their publishing history, and the gradual refinement of the registration system. Thus while the fact of death certification led Farr to devise classificatory systems in the form of nosologies, one of the problems with his nosologies was that they were constructed mainly in terms of a single primary cause. By the turn of the century a more systematic analysis of secondary and tertiary cause of death had been developed, which was of great benefit not only to the medical profession, but also to the life assurance societies.

The developments in epidemiology and vital statistics facilitated by civil registration have been prominent among the relationships between medicine and numbers studied by historians in recent years, but were not unique: several different quantitative approaches were unfolding in Victorian medicine, among which the use of quantitative reasoning in electrotherapy in specialised hospitals for nervous diseases became a controversial issue. John Senior's discussion of electrotherapy shows that electrophyisologists, throughout the century, were occupied with the measurement of minute bioelectric currents in the microcosm against bodily health. Medical men evaluated their electrotherapeutic practices incorporating the whole range of recognised nervous diseases from the organic to the functional, and tables of vital statistics were used in hospital reports to validate the findings of the nervous specialists.

Vital statistics and actuarial methods remained the principal forms of statistics in use in Victorian Britain, and they were primarily applied to medical and governmental purposes. This situation began to change in the 1870s, when Francis Galton began to examine statistical and biological variation, and demonstrated that standardised comparisons could be made by using the law of frequency (the normal distribution). Galton, who was a cousin of Charles Darwin, was one of the last of the Victorian amateur scientists, a veritable empiricist, whose motto was 'count everything that can be counted' – including the efficacy of prayer, the average flush of excitement at horse races, and boredom at meetings.[14] Best known to modern historians as the man driven by Darwinian theory to a quest for the biological foundations of human society, as the originator of eugenics and the author of *Hereditary Genius* (1869), Galton's work on heredity gave scope to many of his statistical innovations. Between 1874 and 1897 he devised the median, probable error and inter-quartile range, and also introduced graphical measures of simple regression and correlation. These techniques found wider application when the Darwinian zoologist, W.F.R. Weldon, began to use them in May 1889.

Eileen Magnello examines the epistemic rupture between vital statistics and mathematical statistics at the end of the nineteenth century. She argues that this arose from the Darwinian biological concepts at the centre of Weldon's statistical and experimental work on marine organisms in Naples and in Plymouth, which gave rise to the development and construction of Pearsonian statistics. Karl Pearson and his students played a key role in the successful adoption of statistics by the medical community in the twentieth century, and Magnello argues further that Pearson's statistical methods provided the framework for Austin Bradford Hill's work on the randomised clinical trial.

Pearson's statistical methods were contentious for many medical practitioners in the early years of the twentieth century. The bacteriologist Almroth Wright, in particular, objected strenuously to Pearson's statistical methods for determining the efficacy of anti-typhoid inoculation. Rosser Matthews examines the debates between Pearson and Wright over the statistical and experimental procedures for measuring the opsonic index, the method developed by Wright for testing the efficacy of inoculation. Yet despite Wright's powerful opposition, and the suspicions aroused in the medical community by Pearson's criticisms of clinical knowledge, the Pearsonian methodology was carried forward into the medical world of the inter-war years by Major Greenwood, and by his protegé Austin Bradford Hill, who successfully extended the use of Pearsonian statistical methods into the wider medical community. Since 1945, the clinical trial has become an integral tool of modern therapeutic and clinical medicine, although one whose methodologies are continually subject to revision and criticism.

For most of the period covered by the essays in this book, the development of the relationship between numbers and medicine, between medicine and quantitative procedures, has been a minority interest, often the subject of apathy or hostility from the wider medical community. The saying that anything can be proved by statistics has been current among British medical men since at least the 1850s, and it was only in the 1890s, against a background of increasing scientific rigour and the emergence of Pearsonian statistics, that members of the English medical community began to recognise that numerical methods might have applications beyond preventive medicine. In 1894, for example, one physician claimed to have discovered a new antidote to prussic acid poisoning, and to have successfully treated forty persons accidentally poisoned with prussic acid. Reporting this story, the *Lancet* noted that most physicians would not meet a case of prussic acid poisoning in a life-time, and that the drug is so powerful that treatment is usually impossible: 'What satisfactory explanation can possibly be suggested for such extensive experience?'[15] Such claims, it was recognised, could not be made if new discoveries were subject to statistical controls. Despite the interest of medical men in quantitative techniques in earlier centuries, it was the acceleration of medical expertise and medical discoveries occurring in the later decades of the nineteenth century that gave impetus to the tighter integration of mathematical statistics with medical research and discovery. It was only after World War II with the medical popularisation of the randomised clinical trial, and with the thalidomide tragedy and world recognition that therapeutic advances must be rigorously monitored and controlled, that mathematical statistics came into its own as an accepted regulator of medical research.

Eileen Magnello
Anne Hardy

Notes

1. See the series 'History of Epidemiology' in *Sozial-nud Präveatirmedizin* 45–46 (2001-02).

2. William Coleman, 'Therapeutic trials in nineteenth century Germany' in Lorenz Krüger, Gerd Gigerenzer and Mary Morgan (eds), *The Probabilistic Revolution. Volume 2. Ideas in the Sciences.* (Massachusetts, 1987), 201–26.

3. Desirée Cox-Maksimov, "The making of the clinical trial in Britain, 1910-1945: Expertise, the state and the public", Ph.D. thesis, Cambridge, 1997.

4. Harry Marks, *The Progress of Experimental Science and Therapeutic Reform in the United States, 1900-1990* (Cambridge: Cambridge University Press, 1997).

5. Edward Higgs, 'A cuckoo in the nest? The origins of civil registration and state medical statistics in England and Wales', *Continuity and Change,* xi (1996), 1–20. J. Rosser Matthews, *Quantification and the Quest for Medical Certainty* (Princeton: Princeton University Press, 1995).

6. Ian Hacking, *The Taming of Chance* (Cambridge: Cambridge University Press, 1990).

7. Ted Porter, *Trust in Numbers: The Pursuit of Objectivity in Science and Public Life* (Princeton: Princeton University Press, 1995).

8. Gerd Gigerenzer, Zeno Swijtink, Theodore Porter, Lorraine Daston, John Beatty and Lorenz Krüger, *The Empire of Chance* (Cambridge: Cambridge University Press, 1989).

9. Theodore Porter, *The Rise of Statistical Thinking 1820-1900* (Princeton: Princeton University Press, 1986).

10. John Sinclair, *The Statistical Account of Scotland drawn up from Communications of the Ministry of Different Parishes.* Vol. XX (Edinburgh, 1798).

11. John Eyler, *Victorian Social Medicine: The Ideas and Methods of William Farr* (Baltimore: Johns Hopkins University Press, 1979),

476.

12. For background material to the formation of the Statistical Society of London see Victor Hilts, *'Aliis exterendum,* or the origins of the Statistical Society of London', *Isis,* ixx (1978), 21–43. Also see Laurence Goldman, 'The origins of British social science: Political economy, natural science and statistics, 1830-35', *Historical Journal,* xxvi (1983), 278–292.

13. See Eyler, *op. cit.* (note 11) Chapter 3; Simon Szreter, 'The GRO and the public health movement in Britain 1837-1914', *Social History of Medicine,* iv (1991), 435–64.

14. The only modern study of Galton's life remains D.W. Forrest, *Francis Galton: The Life and Work of a Victorian Genius* (New York: Taplinger Pub. Co., Inc., 1974).

15. Leader, 'The argument of statistics', *Lancet* (1894), i, 1512-3.

1

Death and Method:
The Rhetorical Space of Seventeenth-Century
Vital Measurement

Philip Kreager

In his recent Bateson Lecture, Professor Skinner remarked on the
degree to which the Renaissance tradition of the art of rhetoric
penetrated seventeenth century philosophical and moral reasoning[1].
The point has also been made in the context of the reform of
scientific method, notably in regard to the work of Francis Bacon.
Bacon studies have shown considerable sympathy for the *ars
eloquentiae*, noting how it came to play an ancillary yet instrumental
role in his epistemology.[2] Skinner, in contrast, adheres to the
distinguished line of contemporary negative assessments, from
Hobbes to Sprat and Locke. These writers were concerned with the
need to establish an agreed vocabulary of evaluative terms for
purposes of inquiry. They were sceptical, to put it mildly, of the
methods and aims of rhetoric textbooks which, in systematically
cultivating tropes and circumlocutions, sought to assist speakers and
writers to blur, and thence to controvert, clear argument. Sprat called
such eloquence 'empty satisfaction'.[3]

Bacon's opinion, however, was more circumspect or, perhaps,
calculated. He drew a line between methods used to present
arguments (including presentations of scientific findings) and those
apt to making natural observations and analysing them.
Conventional rhetorical devices retained their fundamental role in
the former, but were supposed to be banished from the latter.
Traditional textbooks on rhetorical and dialectical method inevitably
encouraged authors to conflate persuasion and inquiry. Bacon
described this tendency as 'vicious and incompetent', and as leading
to mere 'juggleries of words' not productive of new knowledge.[4] John
Graunt, with whose work most of this essay will be concerned, drew
the same line: opposed to men whose aims are to 'write and speak

1

wittily', there are those soberly engaged in productive trades and scientific experiments. In his view, the ratio of the number of wits in a population to what he called men of 'solid and piercing heads' would be a telling index of the greatness of a state.[5]

The *ars eloquentiae* may seem an improbable starting point for a paper on mathematics and medicine. Modern opinion has come down firmly on the side of the Sprats and Lockes. 'Rhetoric' is now widely considered a pejorative term. However, Graunt's *Natural and Political Observations*, long regarded as the beginning of medical and social demography, lies between the two perspectives just outlined. On one side, as I shall show, Graunt's deployment of stock rhetorical devices conforms to the delimited uses Bacon advocated. Of course, whether Graunt set out literally to apply Bacon's dicta on these matters is an open question. What I wish to suggest is that the changing conception of rhetoric as a component of method, and, more particularly, the methods and vocabulary which Bacon devised to resolve this actively contested sixteenth and seventeenth-century issue, provide tools for reading Graunt without which much of the significance of his text is lost. By significance I mean not only his numerical treatment of certain problems but the remarkable influence which Graunt's method has exercised on subsequent vital measurement. The *Observations* reflects not only Bacon's rationalisation of rhetorical methods as 'initiative' and 'magistral', but the potent ambiguities of this formulation.

On the other side, Graunt's essay fits readily into the perspective of Professor Skinner's seventeenth-century philosophical critics of the rhetorical tradition. The *Observations* is in large part an attempt to devise a language and procedures which provide a solution to the following problem: What, if any, agreed meaning can be assigned to the salad of evaluative terms by which causes of death are listed in the London Bills of Mortality? In the *Observations* we find that the interpretation of apparently narrow questions of medical and vital classification, hinging on seemingly imponderable terms like 'aged' or 'toads and snakes', turn out to be *exempla* of a general method. Observation as practised by Graunt is not an unvarnished quantitative recording of facts, but a pattern of inference in which political and natural relationships of the kind that concerned Hobbes and Locke were found to be immanent in certain proportional regularities.

The very oddity to the modern ear of taking seriously the quaint and colloquial terms contained in the Bills of Mortality, let alone attributing immanent relationships to them, should remind us that

2

neither the objects nor the ideas of method in early modern inquiry were quite as we would now make them. The conventions of twentieth-century medical statistics and demography assume that it is possible to apply mathematics to human concerns in a purely formal way. Quantitative observation and inference are one thing. Qualitative approaches, including rhetoric, are another. One can well imagine the astonishment that would greet modern statistical textbooks, like Pressat's *Population Analysis* or Hill's *Principles of Medical Statistics*, if they were reissued with new and central chapters on rhetoric as a key methodology of quantitative research.

The convention in almost all historical studies of early modern population inquiry is to describe quantitative procedures and numerical records of the time using modern terms like 'statistics' and 'data'. This is blatant anachronism. We are now accustomed to the fiction that the models, measures and collational formulae of statistics and demography comprise a formal methodology that generally transcends the vagaries of ordinary language and the conditions of its use. But this fiction only emerged gradually in the two centuries after Graunt. So compelling is this ideal that we find great difficulty understanding how valuable quantitative reasoning about society and its problems could be organised systematically other than as statistics. We lack the vocabulary to transcend the significant break in method and culture that separates us from early modern analysts. This too is a problem which early modern rhetorical methods can help us to correct. As I hope to show, thinking our way around a mental world in which conventions, such as now separate quantitative and qualitative methods, were neither necessary nor obvious, can be a salutary exercise.

•

There are four senses in which it is helpful to consider rhetoric as integral to the method of early modern population arithmetic. First, and trivially, we can find examples in writings such as Graunt's of arguments developed according to conventional literary formulae. Second, beneath this surface there were changes in the concept of method in the course of the seventeenth century, of which Bacon's attempt to deploy rhetoric separately from natural observation and scientific interpretation is an important instance. As Graunt closely followed Bacon's advice on the compilation and analysis of natural histories,[6] it is not surprising that he should also adopt Bacon's framework for presenting such knowledge. Such an approach had the advantage of making his work accessible both to old audiences and new. We shall also note more briefly how changes in the foundations of mathematics during the seventeenth century moved in tandem with the separation of inquiry from methods of presentation; this parallel was an important factor in the sophisticated mathematical attention Graunt's work immediately received.

In other words, although rhetoric textbooks were undoubtedly familiar in the milieu in which Graunt moved, they cannot be our sole or main guide. Their influence was conditioned by the altered position which rhetoric came to have in seventeenth century method. Our third concern, therefore, is not so much with evidence of how conventional rhetoric shaped Graunt's work as with the *Observations* as an example of the redevelopment of rhetoric along significantly new lines. The elementary quantitative devices Graunt employed, like addition and proportion, operate in his text in the same way as elementary literary formulae, carrying out the functions of *comparatio, accumulatio, exemplum, metonymia* and other conventional figures. The issue is not simply that quantification may serve rhetorical purposes, but that even the simplest numerical method contains a rhetorical practice which functions methodically to bring about certain outcomes, and which can be seen at work in the earliest apparently modern attempt at quantitative social inquiry.

The fourth question which arises, then, is consideration of the role of rhetoric in the making of Graunt's arithmetic *as a method*. The *Observations* was recognised by his contemporaries and followers as not just a novel application of number to some topical matters, but as a new way of reasoning of a general and potentially scientific kind. In Section III we turn to the central quantitative figure in Graunt's terminology, the 'accompt'. This analogy or metaphor gave a distinctive structure to the arithmetical tropes which are the elementary building blocks of his argument. How are these elements, which operate simultaneously as arithmetical description and rhetorical amplification, combined to make up 'an accompt'? And how, as they are further developed in the course of his text, do they give Graunt's observations an air of evidence so untroubled that 20th century commentators could assimilate them to later concepts of quantitative empiricism? Graunt's accounting practice effectively mobilised and extended the application of conventional literary formulae in a way that was far from trivial.

I

It was common in rhetoric texts of Graunt's time to group together a number of the most frequently used elocutionary figures under the rubric of 'amplification'. As the term suggests, these figures enlarge upon a theme in order to illustrate, sharpen, and enforce it. Hoskins,[7] whose work was copied by Graunt's contemporaries Blount [8] and Smith,[9] lists five figures under amplification: 'comparison', 'division', 'accumulation', 'progression', and 'intimation'. Finding these figures at work in Graunt's *Observations* is a simple matter.

Of comparison Hoskins observes that arguments become forcible 'when things unequal are compared, and that in similitudes as well as examples'; thus, he compares a widow to a ship, remarking that both ask 'much tackling and sometimes rigging'.[10] The image is as striking as the association is unexpected, whether or not we happen to agree with the sentiment. Likewise, one of Graunt's similes likens death due to the 'French Pox' to the incidence of mortality to 'Toads and Snakes'.[11] There is a natural abhorrence, he remarks, of each, yet apparently few die of either cause. Taking the Mortality Bills at face value in this way, he continues, might well encourage men 'in the intemperate use ... of many common Women'. Graunt advances thence to example, which shows otherwise: only Bills from those parishes known for their brothels (St Giles, St Martins-in-the-Fields) enter deaths to 'Pox', whereas others, for example with hospitals (Kingsland, Southwark), show an excess of deaths to 'ulcers' and 'sores'. The point is driven home by a further use of simile, of a kind sometimes called 'emblem' in rhetoric texts:

> it is not good to let the World be lulled into a security and belief of Impunity by our *Bills*, which we intend shall not be only as *Deaths heads* to put men in mind of their *Mortality*, but also as *Mercurial Statues* to point out the most dangerous waies that lead us into it and misery.

As this example indicates, several rhetorical figures are commonly compounded to make a point.

In Graunt's example of why christenings are underreported in the Mortality Bills,[12] all of the elements of accumulation, division, progression and intimation come to his aid. Of 'division' Hoskins remarks, using a suitable quotation from Bacon, that 'to amplify anything is to break it and make an anatomy of it into several parts'.[13] 'Accumulation' is the heaping up of many terms of praise or accusing', not just in a list, but all tending toward the same side or view of a matter; 'progression' is an accumulation which proceeds from secondary arguments to greater and greater ones.[14] 'Intimation... leaves the collection of greatness to our understanding, by expressing some mark of it'.[15]

Graunt, having demonstrated the numerical deficiency of christenings in some parishes, turns to the question of why this should be the case, and what consequences flow from it.[16] His development of this problem is typical of the way he constructs an argument. First he *divides* the causes into four sorts; treating each in turn, he *accumulates* examples into a *progression* of increasingly greater force, concluding with arguments forcible not only on moral grounds, but carrying legal and financial consequences. The first reason, he says, 'was Religious Opinion against *Baptising of infants,* either as unlawful or unnecessary'. This reason, however, he finds insufficient: the deficiency of the Bills was so great in the period to which he refers (1650-60) that, for the sums recorded to be accurate, the majority of English people would have to have been convinced that baptism was unnecessary. The implication or *intimation* here is that no one could take seriously the possibility that the policies of the Interregnum were widely accepted as legitimate. The second cause to which Graunt refers is ministers' scrupulousness regarding the ability of parents to carry out the demands made in the rite of baptism; having been refused by one minister, such parents would naturally seek out a more lax one, that is, one who 'had not the Authority or Command of the *Register* to enter the Names of the *baptised*'. Graunt's intimation here follows the same line as the preceding. The third cause further blackens our view of any literal reading of the records of the period by suggesting that non-conforming parents were either unwilling or unable to pay the 'little fee' required at registration. In citing the fourth cause, Graunt finally comes to the point of his intimations:

> Upon the whole matter it is most certain, That the number of Heterodox Believers was very great between the said year 1650 and 1660; and so peevish were they, as not to have the Births of their Children *Registered,* although thereby the time of their coming of Age might be known, in respect of such Inheritances as might belong to them; and withal, by such *Registring* it would have appeared unto what *Parish* each Child belonged, in case any of them should happen to want its relief.

There is nothing very surprising in this kind of rhetorical progression on Graunt's part. The elements of rhetoric remained a central part of ordinary schooling in the first half of the seventeenth century.[17] We know of Graunt that he was 'educated while a boy in English learning' and that he later picked up Latin, the locus of the intellectual tradition from which the methods of dialectic and rhetoric came into the mainstream of English education.[18] Graunt's public presence was remarked. Pepys for instance records that in conversation he was a stylist, and Aubrey notes that Graunt was in demand as an arbitrator of trade disputes.[19] As the point of rhetoric is management of the knowledge, opinion and affairs of men, and as Graunt wishes both to demonstrate his new method and to use it to make certain topical arguments, we can only expect that he would avail himself of conventional procedures designed to assist precisely these ends. The real matter which concerns us, however, lies elsewhere: In what sense can seventeenth-century developments in rhetorical method be understood as shaping his novel method of population analysis?

•

Bacon's separation of rhetorical and investigative aspects of inquiry was emphatic, but not categorical. In effect, he recognised that in scientific and scholarly inquiry the door is always open at some stage to rhetorical influence. A good command of tropes, their uses and abuses, is arguably one of the few positive options for maintaining a critical grasp on the potential problems and opportunities this open door presents. Bacon emphasised two contributions of rhetoric to scientific inquiry in particular. They are familiar enough today, even though we no longer consider them matters of rhetoric. And they describe very well the difficulties faced by authors, like Graunt, who need to find ways of introducing new methods and unexpected results.

First, in order for methods and findings to become part of general knowledge, specialists need to be able to transmit them in compelling non-specialist terms. As Bacon said,

> logic [by which he meant the method of the *Novum Organon*] handles reason in truth and nature, and rhetoric handles it as it is planted in the opinion of the vulgar. And therefore Aristotle wisely places rhetoric between logic on one side, and moral and civil knowledge on the other, *as participating in* both ... the proofs and persuasions of rhetoric ought to differ according to auditors (emphasis added).[20]

Graunt's choice of the title for his work, in giving equal weight to the *natural* and *political* character of his observation, signals that his method and findings 'participate in both' scientific inquiry and moral and civil knowledge. As I have noted in detail elsewhere,[21] he did more than just claim that his book was a natural history of the kind Bacon advocated; Graunt's method followed step-by-step the advice Bacon gave on the compilation of natural histories and the critical evaluation of evidence. What Graunt added to Bacon's method derived largely from the moral and civil side of his sources. He drew on two domains familiar to his 'auditors'. First, he inserted commonplace terms and computational procedures of merchant book-keeping into the logic of natural history, as a classificatory and inductive tool. Second, he identified the numerical regularities to which this tool gave rise with the wider political and moral schema of the body politic and the Renaissance distinction of intrinsic and extrinsic value. As it happens, these latter conceits may also be traced to Aristotle.[22]

I shall give examples below to illustrate Graunt's synthesis of numerical and natural historical methods. For the moment, I wish only to call attention to the fact that the joint 'participation' of Graunt's observations in the logic of scientific inquiry and its civil and moral uses is reflected in the rhetorical stance of his text. That is: reflected on the different sets of auditors (or readerships) to which he addressed himself, and how he addressed them. There are, of course, the patrons: the ministers of state and members of the Royal Society who comprised a scientific and political elite. Graunt's images here appropriately match the natural and political character of his observations to the mixed interests and problems of his audience. The Royal Society, in Graunt's epistle dedicatory, becomes the 'parliament of nature'; the intrinsic proportions revealed in his natural history are necessary 'even to balance Parties and Factions in *Church* and *State*'; concluding the essay, he leaves to the discretion of the 'Sovereign and his chief ministers' whether they alone should be allowed access to the methods and findings of population arithmetic.[23]

These formal and obsequious allusions belong to the immediate period of the Restoration. There is, nonetheless, an unmistakable current of tension in the *Observations* which recalls the revolt against absolutism of the immediately preceding period. Knowledge of the number and strength of a people in relation to state revenue and conscription had always been the private prerogative of princes. Yet here is a book, written by a former captain of the 'trayned bands', that proposes an open method for obtaining precisely such information. It was quickly published and widely read. The dedications, in other words, have a large element of royal lip-service in them.

Graunt evidently had considerable respect for his general readership. At several points he remarks that the tables he provides will enable 'all men' to carry out their computations and analyses, that they 'may better understand the hazard they are in' (i.e. from different causes of death) [24] and 'may both correct my *Positions* and raise others of their own'. 'For herein', he continues, 'I have, like a silly School-boy, coming to say my Lesson to the World (that Peevish, and Tetchy Master) brought a bundle of Rods, wherewith to be whip'd for every mistake I have committed'.[25] As we shall see, this openness in Graunt is not just a rhetorical flourish or advertisement, but a calculated stance. On the one hand, the ideas of open presentation Graunt follows are a unifying feature of Bacon's 'initiative' and 'natural historical' methods, which run sharply counter to the covert attitude to evidence assumed in rhetoric textbooks. On the other, this 'open' procedure in fact carries on precisely those blurring and obscuring functions described in rhetoric texts, insinuating a method of analysis and interpretation into topical questions of public, moral and personal policy. The calculations left for completion by the reader are an effective means of making Graunt's method and interpretations appear to be the reader's own; the reader might make his own computations, but the only procedures extant were the ones Graunt had laid down. Such *double entendre* doubtless recommended itself in an era in which new methods and findings raised potential questions not only of political rectitude but heresy. Graunt and Bacon were both wary of such complications.

The second contribution of rhetorical method emphasised by Bacon further blurs the relation between the transmission of knowledge and its conceptualisation. Like the first contribution, the role of rhetoric here is to assist the speaker or writer in addressing diverse audiences. The second use, however, is also described by Bacon as a 'negotiation within ourselves'. His point is again an elaboration on Aristotle:

> the duty and office of Rhetoric, if it be deeply looked into, is no other than to apply and recommend the dictates of reason to imagination in order to excite the appetite and will. For we see that the government of reason is assailed and disordered in three ways; either by the illaqueation of sophisms, which pertains to Logic; or by juggleries of words, which pertain to Rhetoric; or by the violence of the Passions, which pertains to Ethics... yet the nature of man is not so unfortunately built, as that those arts and faculties should have the power to disturb reason, and no power to strengthen and establish it; on the contrary they are of much more use in that way. For the end of logic is to teach a form of argument to secure reason, and not to entrap it; the end likewise of moral philosophy is to

9

procure the affections to fight on the side of reason, and not to invade it; the end of rhetoric is to fill the imagination with observations and images, to second reason, and not to oppress it.[26]

Discreet use of rhetorical methods is critical in explicating 'knowledge which comes altogether new and strange to men's minds'. As Bacon explains, where knowledge has its roots:

> already seated in popular opinions, [the] need [is] but to dispute and prove; whereas those [new forms of knowledge] whose conceits are beyond popular opinions, have a double labour; first to make them understood, and then to prove them; so that they are obliged to have recourse to similitudes and metaphors to convey their meaning.[27]

In short, the problems raised by new forms of knowledge are not just those of clarification and dissemination. An author, in choosing his terms, examples, and formulae inevitably draws analogies and makes comparisons which rely on, yet may controvert, established positions. As particular terms of phrase and metaphors come to be accepted by the author and his readers, so they come to typify and be identified with the nature of the phenomena, and thence with the methods used to reveal them.

•

Bacon's account of the transmission of knowledge seems always to have required interpretation. Sprat and his fellow founders of the Royal Society, including Graunt, apparently took Bacon's writings as their *raison d'être*, even as the Society moved away from the traditions of method to which rhetoric had belonged. Modern commentators, looking at the evident gap between Bacon's doctrinal pronouncements and his practice, are inclined to emphasise his close reading of Machiavelli.[28] There is, after all, an art and a politics to saying one thing whilst doing another, even in the name of science. Two specific links between Graunt's method and Bacon's need to be traced. First, how does Bacon's theory of the transmission of knowledge apply to the presentation of natural histories, and to Graunt's in particular? Second, given the importance Bacon attached to similitude and metaphor, what is their role in Graunt's *Observations*? Is it confined to amplifications, such as the *exemplum* of the 'French Pox', already noted? Or is it integral to his use of number?

Bacon's account of 'the Method of Discourse'[29] begins with his distinction between two principal methods, 'initiative' and 'magistral'. The former is an active part of scientific inquiry, and

10

consists basically in the injunction to present the stages of observation and experiment in a form which enables readers and listeners to examine them independently and critically. Even in naming this method, Bacon cannot resist insinuating an appropriate 'colouring': 'I call that doctrine *initiative* (borrowing the term from sacred ceremonies) which discloses and lays bare the very mysteries of the sciences'. His *intimatio* refers once again to the inhering unity of divine and natural order; scientists, by implication, are like priests charged with the proper revelation of this order.

'Magistral' methods, in contrast, are used to teach established knowledge, and can be doctrinal and even dogmatic. Here 'there is a kind of contract of error between the deliverer and the receiver; for he who delivers knowledge desires to deliver it in such form as may be best believed, and not as may be most conveniently examined; and he who receives knowledge desires present satisfaction, without waiting for due inquiry'. Bacon identifies the magistral method as fit for general audiences, and the initiative for scientific ones.

Such a distinction raise obvious questions about texts which were aimed at both audiences, like Graunt's and Bacon's natural histories. For detailed guidance on initiative methods we have to turn not to Bacon's doctrinal pronouncements on discourse, but to his more pragmatic remarks on how to write natural histories.[30] Graunt's *Observations* adhered closely to Bacon's precepts: first, the quality of evidence is assessed, both as it depends on direct sense perception and on problems of classification and misreporting; second, as far as possible a tabular form is adopted in presenting evidence, so that readers may readily form their own assessments and check subsequent analyses against them; third in writing the history, Graunt proceeds from this review of the evidence to a series of observations which are arranged as a series of questions or particular topics, i.e., a selective comparison and rearrangements of the primary materials which is designed to identify further relationships and possible practical benefits to mankind. Bacon remarked pointedly that there could be no standard form for such groupings, as they depend not only on the nature of the phenomena being explored, but more particularly on the experience of the investigator. Graunt reiterates both of these points. Another aspect of Graunt's topics and his handling of them which accords with Bacon's instructions is as we have seen, his attention to morally suspect topics. Bacon went out of his way to remark in the *Parasceve* that 'things mean, illiberal and filthy' are as much a part of nature as those that are pure; the investigator should seek 'light and information from whatever

11

source'; but he should also strike a balance by interspersing the history with 'general and catholic observations' as appropriate.[31] Finally the tendency to express most any important relationship in the form of a proportion is a general characteristic of the methods of dialectical and rhetoric which shaped both author's presentations. Although Bacon commonly states his inductions in the form of proportional relationships, he does not, like Graunt, give them a numerical expression.[32]

Bacon's assertion of the primacy of the investigator's own experience, when combined with an eagerness for scientific resolution of human problems, provided his followers with ample room for interpretation. It effectively licenses the investigator to reason directly from evidence as he sees it to any realm of human relationships that he thinks knowledge of the evidence will help to improve. Similitude and metaphor, as Bacon said, assist the transmission of new knowledge, and the *comparatio* Graunt draws between nature and society in explicating the incidence of venereal disease is a case in point. The resemblance is made more potent by the fact that the relationship he posits begins as an analogy, but ends in a brute, material lesson: the 'pox' is a physical and mortal suffering which corresponds to a specific moral failing. Simple proportions presented according to the initiative method thus obtain immediately a magistral force.

This transference is not confined to specific instances, but is characteristic of general terms of method which Graunt shared with Bacon. 'Observation', 'accompt' and 'sense' all admit multiple usage: they refer variously to the raw evidence which nature provides; to this evidence as recorded and 'corrected' by analysis, or seemingly immanent in such evidence; and to magistral remarks that may be made on the basis of all of these evidential forms.

This ambiguity was fundamental to Bacon's programme as the Royal Society inherited it. On the one hand, investigators employing appropriate methods were supposed to be able to recognise resemblances in natural phenomena directly. Once such similarities had been observed, it was reasonable to explore possible similarities in other features, and possibly in origins and processes of development underlying them. Certain resemblances appeared, moreover, to unite phenomena belonging to entirely separate fields of inquiry. The expectation or hope in such cases was that similar scientific principles would turn out to govern apparently disparate domains of knowledge. This epistemology provided the basis of some of the most striking rules Bacon put forward. Jardine notes as an example the universal principle he applied at once to physics and politics: 'putrefaction is more contagious before than after maturity'.[33] Clearly such fruits of observation and induction are not rhetorically neutral.

II

We can now turn to a more detailed examination of this use of similitude and metaphor in Graunt's numerical analysis, the 'negotiation' within his text that made his quantitative method not only new and accessible, but forceful and compelling. Graunt did not use arithmetic and number as formal devices, nor merely for computation. In the terms of his own time, his method was a 'mixed mathematics'; close study of his work is of general interest because it enables us to understand this now largely forgotten attitude to mathematical practice.

To begin with, we shall look at one of Graunt's calculations often cited as establishing his pioneering demographic credentials: his attempt to calculate the number of inhabitants of England and Wales and its relation to London's excessive mortality. The very complexity of the sequence of computations Graunt employs on this topic provides ample material with which to disentangle two closely related questions. How could a new and sometimes torturous method of quantitative reasoning be readily accessible to a wide and various audience, most of whom were not mathematicians? And, how was it possible for this approach, despite the fabric of approximations, hypothetical corrections, and sheer guesses on which it was founded, to carry conviction? In Graunt's development of the problem, the rhetorical figures previously noted in his text are once again evident. Here, however, we begin to see that these devices are used not only to elaborate certain moral and political implications arising from sums and proportions dying: arithmetic is itself the prime instrument of rhetorically controlled comparison and amplification.

•

The most frequently reprinted rhetoric manual of the later sixteenth century, Thomas Wilson's *Arte of Rhetorique*, lists 'reckening' amongst its figures, describing it simply as 'when many things are numbered together'.[34] Several of the figures we have already encountered, like *divisio*, *accumulatio* and *progressio* may, as their names suggest, be implicitly quantitative in character. Nowhere, however, do textbooks go so far as to suggest that students might gain persuasive powers by actually carrying out computations, let alone mathematical analysis. The paragon of style in these works remains

Spenser, not Dee, Recorde, or Descartes.

Graunt's *Observations* changed all of this, at least where acceptable styles of essay and commentary on man, nature and society were concerned. His text is quite unapologetic about the long and sinuous chains of quantitative reasoning which are one of its characteristic features. In a typical sequence[35] Graunt calculates the impact of high mortality in London on the numbers of people in the country as a whole. The problem is central to the text, as it draws on calculations made at other points in the argument, and supplies, in turn, the sums and proportions necessary for further computations.

First, Graunt introduces an estimate of London's inhabitants in and outside the walls (460,000 souls) which he says is calculated later in the text. In fact, although he does subsequently provide three different ways of estimating London's inhabitants *within* the walls, he never applies them to those *without*.[36] Nonetheless, he proceeds to use this sum to calculate the number of people in England and Wales: asserting that London contributes 1/15th of the nation's tax revenue, and assuming that people are in general proportional to tax contributions, he multiplies the 460,000 by 14, giving a total of 6,440,000. Curiously, he then subtracts 460,000 from this to get a total for the nation as a whole, less London; he then applies to the resulting sum the fraction $1/7$, which (again referring to calculations later in the text) he says is the proportion of natural increase in the country over 40 years. Although he subsequently provides sums from a single rural parish which can be used to arrive approximately at this multiplier, he never actually calculates it.[37]

The proposed rate of natural increase of 1/7 yields a total of 854,000, over 40 years. Graunt then remarks that London could make good its excess of burials over christenings if only 250,000, or 6,000 persons per annum of this increase, were sent up to the city. The replenishment then works out as follows: the supposed 250,000 is imagined as distributed on a per annum basis over 40 years, according to an estimate of the average number of deaths in an average family (the latter again referring to numbers given elsewhere in the text); this distribution is then compared to series of burials in London over two shorter periods within the 40 years; it turns out that there are approximately 6,000 more deaths than births in these periods, corresponding to the rate of replacement Graunt proposed. Whilst an estimate of average family size and mortality does appear later in the text,[38] these sums and proportions, like Graunt's reference to proportional tax revenues, are not supported by any evidence.

There was no precedent for this sustained piling of proportional

14

calculation on proportional calculation as the basis of a political and moral essay. Even for a modern audience accustomed to quantitative social sciences, Graunt's reasoning requires close attention. Nonetheless, the book was evidently read very widely, going through four editions in as many years, to say nothing of reviews, later editions, dictionary citations, translation, and pamphlets containing pirated extracts.[39] Graunt's 'auditors' ranged from the mathematical elite of Huygens, Halley, De Witt, Leibniz and the Bernoullis, to the minimally numerant, like Pepys. The diversity of his seventeenth and eighteenth-century audience is perhaps best judged by the range of his successors in the writing of population arithmetics. With exceptions, like Halley or Lavoisier, they were not mathematicians and scientists, but merchants (Petty, Davenant), churchmen (Derham, Süssmilch, Brakenridge, Foster, Muret), surveyors and estate managers (Richards, Laurence, Fleetwood), physicians (Short, Haygarth, Mourgue, Blake), and public officials (King, Vauban, Kersseboom, Moheau, Necker). There can be little doubt that Graunt succeeded in what Bacon called the 'double labour' of presenting his new method to a general audience in a way that was both understandable and compelling.

Many of these successors probably did not know Graunt's work in the original. They did not need to. The *Observations* set in motion an art of reasoning, a distinctive mixed mathematics the subject and import of which were accessible to anyone who was literate and possessed a rudimentary awareness of number. More than this, Graunt's essay was immediately recognisable as a contribution to practical mathematics in the wider sense understood at the time.

In the seventeenth century the phrase 'pure mathematics' still referred to geometrical ideals of the old Scholastic curriculum. 'Mixed mathematics', in contrast, described a steadily expanding body of thought and practice addressed to quantity as manifest in the nature of things. Each subject from book-keeping to mechanics was thought to have its own inhering numerical character and logic. Early in the century Bacon had remarked favourably the growth of mixed mathematics, noting that 'there will be more of them, if men not be idle',[40] and in the course of the seventeenth and eighteenth centuries a chorus of mathematical practitioners from Wilkins to Barrow, Arbuthnot and Boyle developed his theme.[41] The prestige of mixed mathematics is noteworthy, as it was not regarded as flowing from developments in pure mathematics (in the way that, for example, statistical applications are today seen as secured ultimately in formal foundations of the calculus of probability). Rather, mixed

15

mathematics stood independently, and in the course of the century exercised a major influence on changing conceptions of the foundations of mathematics. Practical arts which had given rise to particular mixed mathematics, like hydraulics, engineering and even gaming, appeared to provide not only a body of experience in formulating material problems in quantitative terms, but specific techniques of observation and measurement that led to the growth of new forms of pure mathematics.[42] Graunt's *Observations* was in its own time perhaps the most famous of all such contributions.

The 'mix' in Graunt's mixed mathematics owed, as has been said, to his application of an apparently humdrum practical art, book-keeping. But beneath his 'shop-Arithmetic' lay a more fundamental and familiar set of associations: number, reckoning and death as the idiom of the Last Judgement. Graunt's simple similitude was that each death represents a subtraction from the living, an entry in God's or nature's 'accompts'. And just as death displaces a person or soul to some specific immortal 'population', so each christening incorporates a new person or soul into a mortal one. Graunt's chosen point of entry into this old theme was Bacon's *Natural History of Life and Death*. Bacon had argued that men should observe nature in order to discern possible reflections of God's laws; whilst such knowledge was bound to be a pale record of these laws, it nonetheless offered possible guidance on improving individual and collective life. Such a phrasing inevitably suggested that longevity was a kind of measure of man's success in this attempt. Bacon therefore proceeded to recite all the cases of long-lived persons in history of whom he could find a record, carefully noting those aspects of their physical and moral comportment that 'doe signify long life'. Graunt, expressly taking up Bacon's inquiry, likewise adopted Classical images of the symmetry of divine, natural and political order.[43]

Graunt's seventeenth-century 'auditors' would thus not have needed sophisticated mathematical abilities to appreciate the kinds of connections he was trying to make or his general strategy of making them. A minimally numerate reader (say, who had been introduced to arithmetic in school, but never became skilled at it), could have understood Graunt's sums and proportions from their context as descriptive quantitative statements about more or less, increase and decrease, balance and imbalance in man's state. That numerical differences could be telling in trade, war and politics was likewise a commonplace traced to ancient sources. Even rather complicated strings of computations, such as recited above, employ number in a grammatical form which can be read as merely nominal and adjectival ('460,000 Souls'; 'the proportion of 3 dying out of 11 families', 'the *Burials* increase 206 *per Annum*'; etc).

In short, awareness and intelligibility of number do not necessarily depend on computational ability; numeracy is to some extent merely a part of the ordinary language in which many matters, like life and death, can be discussed. It is in this context that the implicitly quantitative character of Hoskins' rhetorical figures ceases to be an incidental matter. When we look at how a logic or method is built up out of recurring use of rhetorical devices, of which numerical representation is but a part, we begin to see how mere quantification came to be invested with a special capability to reveal truths about man and the nature of human society.

•

'How can you commend a thing more acceptably to our attention', Hoskins writes, 'than by telling us it is extraordinary and by showing us that it is evident?' He recommends the most elementary figure in the rhetorician's repertoire, *comparison*, which 'is either of things contrary, equal, or things different'.[44] As we have seen, for Graunt, as Hoskins, contraries provide the most striking figures with which to organise discussion: there are more and more London inhabitants, yet the substantial excess of burials over christenings shows that human numbers in the city should be shrinking. Here is an extraordinary 'thing', a state of affairs contrary to all ordinary expectation, which arouses our interest and begs for explanation. Graunt's method in 'solving' this problem is to *accumulate* a series of numerical comparisons each of which is in itself evident or readily appreciable to ordinary apprehension. Appropriately, he builds up this picture using the simpler forms of comparison Hoskins cites, that is, those relating to things equable or which rely on easily recognisable differences. Let us look again at this passage, this time with the benefit of Hoskins' guidance, placing it within Graunt's usual arithmetical procedure.

Graunt's readers, by the time they have reached Chapter VII (in which the imbalance of burials and christenings is treated), have had ample introduction to the way Graunt treats similar and dissimilar phenomena. In general, 'things equal' or at least similar are added together; 'things different' are compared by means of proportions. Thus, annual series of mortality that behave in the same way (e.g. which are fairly regular from year to year, or are due to related causes) Graunt combines into a single sum or 'accompt'; departures from this pattern, such as plague years, are then compared by means of proportions or ratios which show which years were the worst, or which causes of death were most important relative to the plague. Proportions may, however, also be used to recognise equals, as when Graunt compares changing ratios of 'livergrown', 'rickets', and 'stopping of the stomach' to show that these classifications refer to related causes of death.[45]

Graunt uses the same logic of *comparatio* in treating proportions of christenings to burials. Annual series of mortality for certain years are chosen as a basis for calculation because their regularity or equivalence allows them to be summed over a given duration; supposed migrants to London are assumed to be distributed in equal proportions over time; differences between the unhealthiness of London and the fruitfulness of rural areas is established by comparing proportions of burials to christenings in each; and so on.

Recognising that Graunt's approach is, at its most elemental, an ordered accumulation of quantitative similitudes and differences, is helpful in several respects. First, the seeming complexity of his computation of London's growth can be disentangled into a relatively simple series of comparisons, as follows:

i.   The problem: the proportion of burials to christenings in London indicates a decrease of its people, yet London appears to be expanding, as shown by observation ('its daily increase of Buildings');

ii.   to begin with, Graunt needs some numerical statement of how many people there are in London; he simply postulates a sum which assumes that we accept that his method of calculating inhabitants within the walls holds *pari passu* for those without;

iii.   the total of inhabitants within and without the walls is then assumed to be equally proportionable to their tax contribution;

iv.   the number of burials and christenings in London, and in a rural parish over selected durations, are assumed to be equivalent to the general pattern of births and deaths;

v.   the proportional surplus of christenings in a single rural parish is taken as equivalent to the pool of potential migrants to London;

vi.   the excess of mortality over reproduction in London is observed to be much smaller than the sum given by (v);

vii.   Graunt proposes that London's excess mortality may be assumed to have been distributed equally over a 40 year period;

viii.   the sum calculated in (vii) is equivalent to the sum indicated by (vi), and falls within the proportional rural surplus calculated in (v);

ix.   hence, London's inhabitants lost to excess mortality are replenished from the countryside without seriously undermining the pattern of reproductive surplus in the country as a whole.

Second, we can see from such a listing that the apparent complexity of Graunt's analysis has nothing to do with the arithmetical part of his reasoning. It arises, rather, from the diversity of quantitative 'things' that wind up being treated as similar. The number of inhabitants within and without the walls, their tax contributions, the regularity of their deaths and births at the level of parish, city, family and state, and the choice of durations in which these events occur, all appear as regularly proportionable to each other. Moreover, each numerical expression of this proportionality becomes a potential multiplier which can be used to estimate further balances, as required. Third, the 'contract' between author and reader of which Bacon speaks is assisted by the accumulation of Graunt's lapses: his allusion to other calculations which turn out to be difficult or impossible to find in the text; his habit of abstracting sums now from one part of the Bills or parish records, and now from another, as if the choice of parish or duration was unproblematic; and his repeated interpolation of proportional conjectures. Much of the exercise is in fact a *petitio principii*: it assumes the existence of inhering quantitative regularities which it is the ostensible purpose of his method to demonstrate.

Accumulatio is, in short, the main device of amplification Graunt employs. Unlike the usual compounding of similes described in rhetoric texts, which appeal to visual, historical or other likenesses, Graunt's comparisons rest on a quantitative similitudes and differences interpreted as evidence of inhering properties of nature and society. We can summarise Graunt's arithmetical amplification by saying that similitudes (i.e., comparisons which assert of numerical equivalents) enable him to interpolate hypothetical quantitative relationships into the Bills which they could not in themselves justify; whilst differences (especially proportional comparisons resulting from such substitutions) advance his argument to its next step.

As Jardine[46] remarks more generally of rhetorical presentation, Graunt's observations are put forward as if they formed a logical sequence: a statement of the problem is followed by subsidiary statements which contribute apparently relevant information, and which combine in ways that appear to demonstrate a systematically reasoned conclusion. As the above listing makes clear, however, the sequence is not logical either in the sense of dialectic or syllogistic methods then prevalent, or of statistical inference as would now be expected. Graunt's 'conclusion' is, rather, *intimated* or suggested by the heaping up of proportional relationships to a certain end. 'To support an argument, all that is necessary is that the comparison should be 'apt', that is that it should be fitting to the occasion, and that there should be a large enough degree of resemblance obvious to the reader for him to accept the resemblance as telling'.[47] The ingenuity of Graunt's use of arithmetic for purposes of *intimatio* is that the 'occasion' into which each proportion or similitude fits usually allows the proportion to be read at several levels. His proportions serve as *exempla* of new science; of the progress of mixed mathematics since Bacon; of natural balance inhering in the newly restored body politic; of specific pieces of practical advice arising from the many balances relevant to medicine, trade, and religion that Graunt presents; and, as we shall see, of the internal coherence of merchant book-keeping writ large.

III

As noted earlier, the political context in which Graunt and Bacon wrote made such an overtly conservative stance unavoidable. One of the important outcomes of the preceding analysis, however, is that we can no longer confine the role of rhetoric in the *Observations* to political signposting or moral emphasis. The latter aspects of his method may be called 'rhetorical stance'. Their function is *magistral*, legitimising his observations for various audiences by appropriate allusions to contemporary class structure, to conventional religious values, stock images of the body politic and intrinsic value, or to the prestige of new scientific developments.

Examining Graunt's arithmetic, however, we have seen that his use of rhetoric is not just to insinuate appropriate commentaries into the quantitative regularity of human populations. The second or *initiative* aspect of his method is his use of arithmetic for purposes of rhetorical amplification. Sums and proportions serve Graunt as evidence that apparently extraordinary circumstances are merely natural. Reading the *Observations*, we see that the capacity of rural parishes to sustain the growth of London appears evident in the numbers themselves, provided that a suitably experienced observer has checked their reliability and guided us through the appropriate selection of quantitative similitudes and differences. The numerical product of one series of similitudes and differences may be applied to other series to produce further regularities, and the same may be done with these products in turn. In this way the balance of the body politic is not insinuated but *found* inhering naturally in the pattern of life and death. Simple numerical relations become powerful arguments because particular quantitative descriptions of a few parishes in London and elsewhere are presented as statements about English people in general. In textbook terms, the whole exercise is an extended play not only of *amplificatio*, but of *metonymia*.

A final step in our consideration of Graunt's quantitative method remains. To this point we have considered his arithmetic as a redevelopment of conventional rhetoric, as if quantification was chiefly a vehicle for the selective heaping of similitudes and differences, the better to make compelling arguments. From this perspective arithmetic is just an extension of ideas of quantity available in ordinary language. This perspective is obviously incomplete. Although arithmetical relationships may be arranged in artful verbal heaps, they also have a mathematical structure. We need, in other words, to relate Graunt's use of quantification as a means of rhetorical amplification to the specifically arithmetical method he followed: merchant book-keeping.

The key quantitative figure in Graunt's method is 'the Accompt'.[48] He employs it frequently, and at several levels of analysis. The first thing to note about Graunt's usage is that 'accompt' is yet another metaphor or similitude. The basic analogy is that the London Mortality Bills are like a merchant's books. The presence of this analogy at the root of Graunt's numerical reasoning is particularly important because it reminds us why Graunt's arithmetic cannot be assimilated directly to statistics. Merchant accounting in the seventeenth century was not statistical either in its attitude to the compilation of numerical records, or as a practice dependent on mathematical probability. The analogy was, however, instrumental in opening up a new and extensive range of arithmetical applications for traditional uses of language as codified in rhetorical textbooks. By examining the three main ways in which Graunt uses the term 'accompt', and the set of quantitative procedures that compose them, we can specify more accurately the nature of the legacy which modern quantitative methodologies may trace to his work.

•

At the most general level, Graunt refers to the whole of the London Mortality Bills, and the raw sums in them, as 'an Accompt'; within this, the many annual and weekly series which compose the Bills ('a true Accompt of the *Plague*', 'Accompts of both *Burials* and

21

Christenings, and also of *Weddings* in the Country', and so forth) are also denoted by the term.[49] 'Every *Tuesday* night', Graunt explains, the parish Clerk 'carries in an Accompt of all the *Burials* and *Christenings* happening that Week, to the *Clerk* of the *Hall*. On *Wednesday* the general Accompt is made up and printed, and *Thursday* published and dispersed'.[50] We would now use a number of different terms where Graunt employed just one; his 'accompts' suggest the overlapping entities now called population, data, statistics, enumeration and compilation. None of the latter terms figure in Graunt's working vocabulary.

Graunt's computations, as he says, are based only on a selection of 'those Accompts which have been kept ... in order'; he subjects them to a book-keeper's scrutiny in order to 'correct' misclassification, redundancy, miscounting and other 'neglect', 'errours' or 'confusion in the Accompts' [51]. In usual merchant practice, book-keepers first entered transactions as they occurred into a day book, later transcribing this rough register into ledgers where each item was tabulated in its correct category or series of transaction. Thus Graunt, from the 'gross' or 'general accompts' provided in the bills, separates 'Accompts of *Epidemical Diseases*' from those of '*Chronical*' ones, and tables of 'notorious diseases' (like 'rupture', 'leprosie' or 'suddenly') from 'casualties' (including death to physical accidents and circumstances like 'shot', 'starved', 'drowned', etc.). He often merely reports the sums and products of his tables, as when he simplifies a menagerie of categories including 'teeth', 'overlaid', 'convulsion', and 'worms' under the heading 'childrens diseases'.[52] His grouping of 'French Pox', 'ulcers' and 'sores', already noted, is another example.

Graunt's 'corrections' also follow merchant practice, by using proportional checks to ensure the relative accuracy of series. In contemporary double entry book-keeping, each transaction was recorded in matching columns of 'debtor' and 'creditor'; tables could then be examined very quickly both to find the changing state of balance and imbalance between columns, but also as a check on computational errors. Thus Graunt, on finding that two series of plague deaths do not maintain consistent proportions over time, goes back along the series and, having located an irregularity, inserts proportional adjustments so that both series as a whole exhibit the same regularity that they maintain in most periods.[53]

The first sense in which we may understand Graunt's use of 'accompt', therefore, refers to general accounting practice: the set of accepted procedures which order sums and transactions as a structure of categories, together with the proportional checks used to maintain numerical consistency within and between them. Graunt's application of the accounting model was not, however, confined to routine procedures for compiling, correcting and tidying the Bills. The second sense of 'accompt' refers to methods of inquiry. It is here that the difference between his accounting model and statistics is most evident. Graunt's calculations are not of populations, rates and trends as now understood, but of 'trial balances'.

Historians of accounting practice have observed that the provision of trial balances was one of the main objectives of successful merchant book-keeping.[54] Seventeenth-century accounting practice did not use merchants' books to calculate total wealth or to forecast trends. In other words, there is no analogue to be found between 'population' as now used in statistics and a merchant's total capital. To evaluate a given transaction, merchants compared the state of debt and credit in the specific accounts relevant to it, taking into consideration proportional affects of interest, insurance and other expenses on those accounts, and, where necessary, introducing appropriate *ad hoc* proportional guesses as multipliers to allow for pending transactions or other pieces of information not at the moment available. The calculation was worked out in terms of proportions of debt and credit at a certain time or in a limited duration relevant to the given transaction. The 'true accompt' of each deal, that is, the real profit or point of a transaction, was better indicated by these provisional estimates than by attempting to make more abstract calculations of a given sale or purchase as a function of the merchant's total worth or the trend of his business as a whole.

Graunt reflects this pragmatism in the sums he uses as denominators in his calculations. Demographers now construct indices so that they may be expressed as functions of a single standardised population which appears as the denominator of a given rate or rates. Comparison of rates from different populations usually requires that their parameters are all defined in the same way. Graunt's long chains of proportional reasoning, however, commonly employ not one but a half a dozen different 'populations', which differ not only in composition but duration. As noted in the case of London's surplus mortality, there is first an unexplained total of 460,000 Londoners, from which further proportional estimates are generated of the 6,440,000 English and Welsh, and the 5,980,000 non-Londoners. The central issue in his calculation – the surplus in the balance of burials to christenings per annum over 40 years – depends only partially on these totals. It is calculated by comparing two other 'populations': the total burials for London in two series, dated 1603-1612 and 1635-1644; and the increase in the number of people in the country outside of London (i.e., the 5,980,000 multiplied by 1/7, or the proportional increase observed in a single Hampshire parish in the period 1569-1588). The comparison of these totals is supposed to confirm Graunt's estimate of 460,000; however, they require yet another 'population' (Graunt's conjecture of the number of London families) before the calculation can be completed. Graunt's reasoning may be summarised by saying that the point of his arithmetical method is not the modern demographic objective of standardisation; the method of trial balances proceeds, rather, by devising a number of semi-independent chains of proportional reasoning, in the hope that all will wind up in more or less the same result.[55]

•

At this point rhetorical figures like *comparatio* and *accumulatio* plainly cease to be sufficient in themselves to understanding how the fabric of Graunt's observations is gradually built up. Yet we should be wary of leaping to the conclusion that the introduction of numerical and observational methods enables scientific inquiry to cut itself free from rhetorical influence. To the contrary, the methical character of Graunt's accounting arithmetic provides a new and powerful means of mobilising conventional rhetorical devices, giving them not only new 'things contrary, equal or ... different' to compare and accumulate, but a new and inter-related set of proportional devices with which to do so.

This power owes to the close alignment of the three methods which Graunt synthesises in his *Observations*. In short, the steps leading to trial balances are homologous with the stages of observation and induction in natural history, and are laid out according to Bacon's initiative method. The chains of proportions that make up these steps or stages are likewise homologous with the comparisons which make up rhetorical accumulation. This is, however, an *accumulatio* with a difference, since it is guided not simply by the magistral ends to which the argument is headed, but by decisions as to which proportional devices drawn from the repertoire of accounting arithmetic are apt to composing each of the specific trial balances/*exempla* Graunt is developing.

The capacity of accounting arithmetic to augment traditional rhetoric is most easily seen in the diverse meanings or uses of proportion in Graunt's analysis. Ultimately the way arithmetical and rhetorical functions are united in particular proportions enables Graunt to substitute invented figures for numerical evidence. The *Observations*, in other words, is not founded on the 'data' which the London Mortality Bills afford, but, as Graunt insisted, on the intrinsic proportionalities which his method elaborates.[56]

The array of tropes and figures compiled at great length by Hoskins and his fellow rhetoricians contains no devices for extending and modifying meaning that work in precisely the manner of Graunt's main uses of proportion, i.e. as multipliers, corrections and trial balances. Yet there is nothing to keep Graunt's handling of numerical proportions from serving the verbal functions described as *comparatio* and *accumulatio*. A proportion, in other words, may serve the purposes of analogy even though the things compared are not the same at every point. The subtle shifts in meaning that occur may be illustrated by examining Graunt's use of proportion in relation to Hoskins' three part definition of comparison (i.e. of 'things contrary, equal, or ... different': see note 44).

First, in his *comparatio* of London's burials and rural baptisms, Graunt parcels out deaths over a given duration as if they were the same in each year, the proportions serving to show that over time the two series are of 'things equal'. There is nothing, however, in Hoskins' repertoire of figures that captures the essential feature of this equalisation, namely, that it is a distribution. Second, when Graunt 'corrects' a series of plague deaths proportionally by increasing or decreasing sums for particular years, he does so in part to sharpen his evidence of 'things different', i.e. that some plague years are radically more dangerous to life than others. Yet Hoskins does not provide us with a vocabulary to describe the way this procedure variously discounts, augments, redistributes, and otherwise alters the significance of particular categories of life and death. Finally, Graunt's reference to certain proportions as the 'hazard' or odds of dying of one disease as opposed to another would certainly count as a powerful device for illustrating 'things contrary'; but analogies to gaming (let alone mathematical probability) are not even intimated by Hoskins and his successors.[57]

Just because rhetoricians of the sixteenth and seventeenth centuries failed to appreciate fully the persuasive power of analogy and proportion in these specific quantitative forms is no reason why we should ignore Graunt's artful development of them. As Graunt shows, the same proportional procedure may produce different rhetorical effects, according to the series to which it is applied. In calculating 'hazard', for instance, he usually takes the total deaths to a specific cause as a proportion of a larger 'accompt' to which he has also assigned them. The significance of 'accompts of men that made away with themselves', or of the 'Accompt of the Green sickness' is, for instance, indicated by the sums of these series as a proportion of the total number of *'Chronical* distempers'. When Graunt adds together several accounts to create a new one, like the proportions dying of 'childhood diseases', he assesses it in the same way. The significance of 'hazard' in the latter case, however, is of a very different order, as he shows in his very first observation. Deaths to childhood diseases are there compared to the plague; the former turn out to be more than four times greater than the latter.[58]

Once again, Graunt's initiative style of presentation sets out the successive stages of observation and induction in a way that appears to allow the reader to think independently. It makes no difference whether we consider these stages as applications of natural history or accounting arithmetic: the arithmetical products of the exercise enable an initiative presentation to end in a magistral argument in which the force of several levels of implication – natural, medical and moral – is compounded in a single numerical *comparatio*.

In the end, Graunt's arithmetical development of *comparatio* and *accumulatio* comes to play a role in his method which parallels and mimics the evidence of the Bills. As we have noted, some summary proportions in Graunt's analysis, like the accompt of the number of families, are not supported by evidence. The absence of actual observations in the Bills, parish records, or elsewhere does not, however, mean that the role of such hypothetical accompts is correspondingly modest. Graunt's guess that on average 3 persons die per 11 families in any given year provides the multiplier on which his analysis of London's excess mortality depends. Whether supported by evidence or not, the function of such proportions is the same: they enable a complex series of events to be expressed in the concise form of a single trial balance which can then be used as a multiplier, factor or variable in subsequent analysis.

Indeed, 'trial balance' is a good translation into accounting parlance of the 'aptness' of rhetorical comparison remarked by Jardine (see note 47). Paraphrasing her remark, we can say that Graunt, in choosing a specific multiplier or ratio with which to correct a given series or to compare it with another, is in effect hunting for a proportion which is 'fitting to the occasion'. The 'occasion' is the numerical similitude/difference he wishes to explore between two or more series and the multiple levels of magistral implication they articulate. The proportion he then calculates is 'apt' because the correction, distribution or other arithmetical relationship it effects shows 'a large enough degree of resemblance obvious to the reader for him to accept the resemblance as telling'.

IV

This paper began with the proposition that the transitional state of rhetoric in the seventeenth century was instrumental to the first population arithmetic. Graunt's *Observations* is shot through with rhetorical devices, which have been summarised under two related heads: 1. arithmetical amplification (in which accounting arithmetic implicitly redevelops and extends devices like *comparatio* and *accumulatio*); and 2. rhetorical stance (in which such similitudes and differences constitute natural, political and moral relationships of wider significance). Graunt made effective use of accounting arithmetic both as a way of giving a quantitative structure to natural history, and for transmitting knowledge according to Bacon's initiative and magistral methods of presentation.

His third use of 'accompt' is, appropriately, as a term of reference for this whole mixed mathematical approach. To some extent this usage reflects the fact that in the seventeenth century, as today, accounting practice was a common metaphor or synomym for explanation. To 'give an account' was to indicate the reason why something was the case. Graunt remarks, for example, in respect of the small number of murders recorded in the Bills, that the leaders of the Interregnum preferred not to carry out public executions 'on Accompt of disturbing their Innovations'.[59] Referring more specifically to his own method, Graunt used 'accompt' as a term for the coherence or proportional regularity which his observations revealed as an inherent property of the Bills. 'A true Accompt of the *Plague*', as he says in his opening index or outline, 'cannot be kept without the Accompt of other *Diseases*').[60] Similarly, the inhering proportional regularity of his accompts contains lessons for the structure of economy and state. The relatively small number of 'starved', for instance, leads to a discussion of public welfare, and becomes a 'little hint' or 'model of the greatest work in the World, which is the making of *England* as considerable for Trade as *Holland*'.[61] More generally, Graunt presents his work simply as 'a true Accompt of people'.[62]

By way of conclusion, it may be helpful to step back from the detail of Graunt's language and method, and consider the implications of his mixed mathematics in the long term. In general, quantitative methods are now thought to gain influence by bringing mathematical analysis to bear on events and relations, systematically clarifying their nature, and enabling us to recognise new patterns in events, and possibly whole new fields of relationships. We should not neglect, however, to ask how events and relations are understood before such analysis gets going. We tend to forget that quantification and simple uses of number are a part of ordinary language as well as of mathematics. Many topics to which mathematics has never been applied systematically are commonly described in terms of quantitative ideas (proportion, more or less, odds, etc.) and numbers which indicate relative magnitude without necessitating computation or algebra. These uses are often inscribed in conventional descriptions of social problems and relationships. The ebb and flow of vital events in Graunt's time is to some extent simply one case in point.

Such conventions do not disappear when mathematical analysis begins, or as it develops. To the contrary, as they are generally accepted in the description of particular topics, events and relations, they are likely to shape people's perception of the aptness of new and more sophisticated mathematical representations. In this way conventional verbal arithmetics, like the uses of similitude and metaphor which Bacon remarked, remain *internal* to the design and gradual working out of mathematical methods as well as part of wider collective representations in society. Ordinary language and existing social conventions are likely to be influenced, in turn, by new mathematical developments. Subsequent practice will continue to employ old general quantitative metaphors and similitudes as vehicles for presenting, interpreting, and understanding the results of arithmetical and higher levels of applied mathematics even as this process continues to alter such conventional descriptions.

The *Observations* enables us to examine this process at a very early stage when the language and assumptions of medical and social statistics, and demography, had yet to be conceived. Graunt's use of proportion simultaneously as a vehicle for *comparatio* and the working out trial balances of life and death shows how new quantitative developments are enmeshed not only in old forms but old *methods* of expression, relying on them whilst also subtly changing their meaning. The ready acceptance and influence of Graunt's method (and probably of most mathematical methods in social inquiry ever since) would appear to owe as much or more to its ability to inform existing orders of knowledge (confirming and rationalising conventions, accommodating new pieces of information, etc.) as to the promise of a new and different basis of knowledge which it appeared to open up.

This approach to Graunt's arithmetic provides a framework within which we can begin to account for the impact of successive mathematical redescriptions of vital events and relations. Graunt's legacy is not only that his *Observations* provided a mixed mathematics of perennially important vital, social and economic matters, but that, following Bacon, it established criteria for assessing and revising any such method. Despite Graunt's rhetorical stance, which directed his readers to interpret certain topics in certain politic ways, his *Observations* was open to critical scrutiny as the methods of initiative presentation and natural history prescribed. The mere carrying out of enumeration, summation, and proportionalisation provided a body of materials to which other verbal arithmetics, as well as other techniques of calculation and analysis, could be applied. The way was opened for other mixed mathematical structures to be built on the Mortality Bills, or on other quantitative sources, employing analogies other than the accounting model Graunt himself followed. This possibility is implicit in Graunt's practice of estimating trial balances by calculations based on alternative assumptions. Just as some of these alternatives were more persuasive than others, so the incremental process began by which the power of one mixed mathematical mode of representation grows relative to others, as certain quantitative phrasings appear better able to clarify relationships in question. Successive formulations in this interpretative process feed back not just into conventional social description, but into the image and nature of the methods themselves.

Graunt's *Observations* acquired in his own lifetime a general reputation under a phrase he did not invent. What Petty called 'political arithmetic' needs to be examined for the changes it introduced into Graunt's method. As population arithmetic evolved in the seventeenth, eighteenth and early-nineteenth centuries, a loosely related set of mixed mathematics, addressed variously to annuity calculations, proofs of divine order, the efficacy of medical practices, *polizeiwissenschaft* and, finally, vital statistics, introduced further methodological differences. Curiously, many of the early-nineteenth century advocates of the newly named mixed mathematics known as 'statistics' argued vehemently that their method was entirely opposed to political arithmetic.[63] Twentieth-century statisticians have then reversed this view, arguing for a slow but effectively seamless continuity of analytical refinement from Graunt's 'statistics' to our own.

Enough has been said here to dispel the mirage that Graunt's 'critical apparatus was a characteristically statistical one'.[64] Whilst the genealogy of population arithmetics after Graunt lies outside the remit of this paper, we can, I think, reasonably apply what we have learned about Graunt's method to the question of how he managed to persuade a long and distinguished line of demographers, statisticians and historians of quantification, from Pearson and Westergaard to the Dupâquiers, that his work was in essence statistical. The answer, of course, is that Graunt did nothing of the kind. These commentators persuaded themselves.

Just how they could succeed in this imaginary exercise is now, however, plain. Twentieth century statisticians brought current ideas of formal methodology and its vocabulary to bear on Graunt's text, concentrating on the similarities they could find between their mathematics and his. The 'mere' presence of enumeration, summation and proportion, noted above, means that any number of quantitative structures may be applied to a given compilation; whether these are recognised or not by the compilers and first analysts, such structures can always be 'found' by later investigators experienced in their own methods and associated verbal arithmetics. In other words, modern commentators have been able to 'find' abstract statistical concepts, the life table, and a variety of techniques for data assessment in the *Observations*, in the same manner that Graunt discovered many things that reflect the preoccupations of learned men in his own time: confirmation of miasmatic theories of disease transmission (in the differing mortality of towns and parishes); evidence of divine disapproval of polygamy (in the balance of the sexes); justification of mercantile arguments concerning the balance of trade (in the geographical movement of populations); and so forth.

In the end, the difference between Professor Skinner's seventeenth century critics of the *ars eloquentiae* and Bacon's complicit use of these arts may not be very great. Sprat sought to banish the eloquence of the 'scholemen' from the new science, but Bacon's understanding of their methods was more profound. The role and function of rhetoric is not only to disguise, but to do so in a way that the methods one employs to that end are also disguised. Whether we banish rhetoric from discussion (leaving it free to operate within our methods without sustained scrutiny) or use it selectively to enforce findings we consider valid, the effect is the same: the workings of rhetoric are concealed, or at least we are deprived of systematic procedures for discerning them. Graunt shared in Bacon's complicity on this score, and the mathematics of population, following his approach, has remained largely complicit ever since.

•

I would like to thank Robert Carver for sharing his notes on Professor Skinner's lecture, and the Wellcome Trust for support during the period in which an earlier draft of this paper was written.

Notes

1. Quentin Skinner, 'Moral ambiguity and the renaissance art of eloquence', F.W. Bateson Lecture, Oxford, 16 February, 1994.

2. Paulo Rossi, *Francis Bacon: From Magic to Science*, trans. S. Rabinovitch, (London: Routledge and Kegan Paul, 1968); Lisa Jardine, *Francis Bacon: Discovery and the Art of Discourse*, (Cambridge: Cambridge University Press, 1974).

3. Thomas Sprat, *The History of the Royal Society of London*, (London, 1667), 17.

4. Francis Bacon, *Of the Dignity and Advancement of Learning, Works*, Vol. IV, ed. J. Spedding, R.L. Ellis and D.D. Heath, (London: Longman, 1858), 410, 455.

5. John Graunt, *Natural and Political Observations*, (London, 1662). References in this paper are to the edition by Charles Henry Hull, ed., *The Economic Writings of Sir W. Petty*, (Cambridge: Cambridge University Press: 1899), Vol II. 324, 396.

6. Philip Kreager, 'New Light on Graunt', *Population Studies*, 42 (1988), 129–140: 130–33.

7. J. Hoskins, *Directions for Speech and Style*, ed. H.H. Hudson, (Princeton: Princeton University Press, 1935).

8. T. Blount, *Academy of Eloquence* (London: 1654).

9. J. Smith, *Mysterie of Rhetorique Unvail'd*, (London: 1657).

10. Hoskins, *op. cit.* (note 7), 18.

11. Graunt, *op. cit.* (note 5), 355–6.

12. *Ibid.*, 361–3.

13. Hoskins, *op. cit.* (note 7), 22.

14. *Ibid.*, 24.

15. *Ibid.*, 25–6.

16. Graunt, *op. cit.* (note 5), 362–3.

17. F. Watson, *The English Grammar Schools to 1660*, (Cambridge: Cambridge University Press, 1908); L. Stone, 'Literacy and education in England, 1640-1900', *Past and Present* 42 (1969), 69, 139.

18. A. Wood, *Athenae Oxoniensis*, Vol. I., no. 711 (London, 1813).

19. Samuel Pepys, *The Diary of Samuel Pepys*, ed. R. Latham and W. Mathews, Vol. IV, 22 (Jan. 1662) and Vol. V, 112 (Jan, 1664)

(London: Bell and Hyman, 1970-83); John Aubrey, *Brief Lives*, ed. A. Clark (Oxford: Clarendon Press, 1898), 271–4.

20. Bacon, *op. cit.* (note 4), 457.

21. Kreager, *op. cit.* (note 6).

22. The distinction between intrinsic value (arising from nature) and extrinsic value (arising from exchange) occurs in the course of Aristotle's discussion of the household. See Aristotle, *The Politics*, ed. and trans. E. Barker, (Oxford: Clarendon Press, 1946), 18–27); on this distinction in merchant writings in the seventeenth century, see Joyce Appleby, *Economic Thought and Ideology in Seventeenth-Century England*, (Princeton: Princeton University Press, 1978), esp. chapter 11.

23. Graunt, *op. cit.* (note 5), 323, 397.

24. *Ibid.*, 350

25. *Ibid.*, 334.

26. Bacon, *op. cit.* (note 4), 455–6.

27. *Ibid.*, 452.

28. Jardine, *op. cit.* (note 2), 163–8, 247.

29. Bacon, *op. cit.* (note 4), 449.

30. Bacon, *Parasceve*, in *Works*, Vol. IV, 251, 271; the remainder of this paragraph is a short summary of Graunt's adaptation of Baconian natural history, detailed elsewhere [Kreager, *op. cit.* (note 6), 130–3].

31. Bacon, *op. cit.* (note 30), 258.

32. Bacon, *Valerius Terminus*, in *Works*, Vol. III, 237; Bacon, *Parasceve*, 259. The importance of proportion in Graunt's and Bacon's works points to the relation between methods of rhetoric and mathematics in the Scholastic curriculum (see. note 42).

33. Jardine, *op. cit.* (note 2), 200. At times Bacon enjoins the drawing of moral and practical lessons from natural history (e.g. in the *History of Life and Death*, in *Works*, Vol. V, 320, 335) and at others explicitly rejects it (e.g. *Parasceve*, 254, 259). The list of conventional figures of rhetoric Graunt employs to joint initiative and magistral effect could be greatly extended if space permitted. An example is the use of one of Bacon's favourite devices, 'aphorisms', which are supposed to be pithy and memorable summary statements of relationships, commonly relying on proportions and analogies. Thus Graunt resumes the seasonality of vital events, saying that 'the more sickly the years are, the less fecund or fruitful of Children also they be', [*op. cit.* (note 5), 368]; or in respect of public welfare, that 'few starve of the many that beg', 320.

34. Thomas Wilson, *Arte of Rhetorique* (London, 1560), ed. G. H. Mair (Oxford: Clarendon Press, 1909), 206. Also see R. A. Lanham, *A*

Handlist of Rhetorical Terms, (Oxford, 1991).

35. Graunt, *op. cit.* (note 5), 369–71.

36. *Ibid.*, 383–5.

37. *Ibid.*, 389.

38. *Ibid.*, 385.

39. The first and anonymous review appeared as 'Natural and political observations made upon the bills of mortality by John Graunt', *Le Journal des Savans* 31 (1666), 613–18; Hull *The Economic Writings of Sir William Petty*, notes further editions of the *Observations* appearing in 1676 and 1759, and a German translation in 1702 (317–8); excerpts from the *Observations* appeared as part of the anonymous *A Collection of Very Valuable and Scarce Pieces Relating to the Last Plague in the Year 1665*, London, 1721; R. Rolt included an entry for 'political arithmetic' in his *A New Dictionary of Trade and Commerce* (London 1761), in which he discusses 'Grant', amongst others; E. Hatton's textbook *An Intire System of Arithmetic* (London, 1731) contains an entry for 'political arithmetic' which, in addition to citing Graunt and others, presents problems in the manner of a primer ('To Find the Number of People by the Coals Imported'; 'To Find the Number of Houses within the Bills'; etc.).

40. Bacon, *op. cit.* (note 4), n. 4, 371.

41. John Wilkins, *Mathematicall Magick*, (London, 1648); Isaac Barrow, *The Usefulness of Mathematical Learning Explained and Demonstrated*, (London, 1734) [from lectures first given in the period 1664-9]; John Arbuthnot, *An Essay on the Usefulness of Mathematical Learning*, (Oxford, 1701); Robert Boyle, 'Of the usefulness of mathematicks to natural philosophy', in *Works*, Vol. 3, 156–62.

42. On the role of practical arts as a stimulus to early modern science, see Rossi, *Francis Bacon*, Ch. I. With reference to specifically mathematical developments, the following very brief summary and example may perhaps suffice. One of the ways in which 'method' came to be a term for rhetoric was by analogy to geometrical proofs; geometry and rhetoric were both pillars of the Scholastic curriculum, and by the 16th century the former had come to be seen as an exemplar of presentation which rhetoric might follow. In geometry, arguments were presented as proofs, i.e. logical series of premises, deductions and corollaries in which each step in the development was laid out and shown either to follow from the preceding or to be justified by reference to other proofs. Rhetoric, whilst not actually effecting proofs, might emulate the form of geometric presentation. In the seventeenth century, however, just as Bacon and his followers rejected rhetoric as a basis of inquiry, so mathematicians came to

question the model of proofs as foundational to mathematical practice. 'New analysis' (i.e. based on algebra) was recognised as more flexible in particular mixed mathematical applications, and more productive of new mathematical ideas, than the 'old' geometric model. Halley's development of Graunt's mixed mathematics of mortality at different ages was typical of this trend: beginning from arithmetical examples, he explored an new probabilistic algebra of death, introducing his geometrical proof only at the end of the paper; the proof functions as a formal generalisation, not as a working part of the inquiry.

43. Kreager, *op. cit.* (note 6), 137–40.
44. Hoskins, *op. cit.* (note 7), 17.
45. Graunt, *op. cit.* (note 5), 357–9.
46. Jardine, *op. cit.* (note 2), 228.
47. *Ibid.*, 196.
48. Kreager, *op. cit.* (note 6), 133–7.
49. Graunt, *op. cit.* (note 5), 327, 333, 388.
50. *Ibid.*, 346.
51. *Ibid.*, 328, 363, 365, 366.
52. *Ibid.*, 349-51.
53. *Ibid.*, 365.
54. B. Yamey, H.C. Edey, and H.W. Thomson, *Accounting in England and Scotland, 1543-1800*, (London: Pitman, 1963).
55. The problem-oriented nature of merchant accounting helps to explain many other features of Graunt's analysis which may appear surprising from a statistical point of view. Graunt, for example, was not troubled by the fact that he gives conflicting proportional estimates of the same account at different points in his text. For instance, in the case of 'aged', the proportion of Londoners surviving age 70 is given as 7/100 [*op. cit.* (note 5), 352], but subsequently Graunt says that only 6/100 survive to age 56; 387. As it happens these proportions refer to slightly different general accounts, one being proportional to 'total casualties', and the other to a hypothetical number based in part on 'total casualties'. The reliance of political arithmeticians on a method based initially on the logic of trial balances has important implications for the contentious nature of their findings, and their difficulty in resolving the priority of different modes of calculation.
56. Graunt, *op. cit.* (note 5), 395: 'Now the foundation of this honest harmless policy is to understand the Land, and the hands of the Territory, according to all their intrinsick and accidental differences.'
57. Graunt, *op. cit.* (note 5), 350. Graunt's approach to 'hazard' differed

as well from the early algebra of probability developed in the period 1655-1672 by Huygens, Pascal and others. See Philip Kreager, 'Histories of Demography: A Review Article', *Population Studies* 47 (1993), 519–39.

58. Graunt, *op. cit.* (note 5), 349.
59. *Ibid.*, 354.
60. *Ibid.*, 332, 353–4.
61. *Ibid.*, 354.
62. *Ibid.*, 332.
63. For example, Jean Peuchet, *Statistique Eléméntaire de la France*, (Paris, 1805).
64. David V. Glass, 'John Graunt and his natural and political observations', *Proc. of the Royal Society* B 159 (1963), 2-32. It would be invidious to single out Glass on this score. Typical citations of Graunt include: 'The first... and extremely competent attempt to draw scientific conclusions from statistical data' (Ian Sutherland, 'John Graunt: a tercentenary tribute', *Jrnl. of the Royal Statistical Society*, A 126 (1963), 537–556); Graunt '... implicitly accepts the stability of statistical ratios', (Karl Pearson, *The History of Statistics in the 17th and 18th Centuries*, ed. Egon Pearson, (London: Griffin, 1978), 30); 'it became possible for a Graunt or a Petty to look at the data as data' (Ian Hacking, *The Emergence of Probability*, (Cambridge: Cambridge University Press, 1991, 106); Graunt has been called variously the 'founder' (cf. Glass) and 'father of demography' (Jacques et Michel Dupâquier, *Histoire de la Demographie* (Paris: Perrin, 1985), 137. In saying that Graunt began the traditions of quantitative description and analysis that we now call demography and statistics, we need to keep in mind not only that he initiated quantitative modes of reasoning that embrace some concepts and procedures that practitioners today recognise, but also those rhetorical devices which remain integral to constructing and interpreting human populations.

2

'The Merchant's Logick': Numerical Debates over Smallpox Inoculation in Eighteenth-Century England

Andrea Rusnock

In 1722 smallpox swept through England causing death, disfigurement and despair. Thomas Nettleton (1683–1742), a physician working in Halifax, Yorkshire, became desperate in the face of tragedy. The suffering of his patients, despite his best efforts at therapy, spurred him to adopt a radical course. Having read reports of smallpox inoculation in the *Philosophical Transactions*, Nettleton decided to try it because inoculation, it was generally agreed, would give patients lifelong immunity. The procedure involved making a small incision on a patient's limb and inserting pus taken from a smallpox pock; a mild case of smallpox typically resulted, but not always. In some instances, patients died from a severe case of smallpox brought on by inoculation. There also was evidence that inoculated smallpox was contagious. These hazards, death and spreading of the infection, were well-known in England from published reports. But did the benefit of immunity outweigh the risks of injury? Nettleton and his contemporaries wrestled with the issue of how to evaluate the new practice of smallpox inoculation.[1]

For his part, Nettleton thought that the only way to establish *'That the Ingrafted Small Pox is far less dangerous than the Naturall'* would be 'by making a Comparison so far as our Experience will extend'. To this end, he conducted a survey of the incidence of smallpox in Halifax and neighbouring towns and tallied how many individuals had contracted it and of those, how many had died. Of the 61 inoculations he had performed by the end of 1722, he recorded only one fatality. His total figures indicated that one-fifth of those who contracted natural smallpox died, while 1 in 60 died from inoculated smallpox.[2]

But how to convince others to undergo inoculation? Would the difference in odds be sufficient to persuade individuals to take the risk? And how should the physician, indeed the community, cope with inoculation gone awry? Nettleton, working alone in a provincial community, developed his own rationale. 'Whenever any shall happen to miscarry under this Operation', he wrote, 'that will indeed be very unfortunate & ill, but in this Case You will have recourse to the Merchants Logick: state the Account of Profitt & Loss to find on which side the Ballance lyes with respect to the Publick, & form a Judgement accordingly.'[3] Nettleton's reason for accepting the risks of inoculation – 'the Merchant's Logick' – introduced a startlingly new type of argument into medicine. It balanced public benefit with personal risk and asked the physician to weigh the welfare of a population against the health of an individual. Merchant's logic argued that physicians should calculate the utility of particular practices by summing up the costs and benefits among a population of patients.

Nettleton was not idiosyncratic in his thought. Various forms of merchant's logic crop up in eighteenth-century medical literature, especially works addressing smallpox inoculation. It was a highly contentious practice and the community divided in its opinion along religious, ethical, and political lines.[4] Mathematical arguments such as those advocated by Nettleton played a central role precisely because they sidestepped these quarrelsome concerns. Beginning in the 1720s, widespread debate both within the medical community and in society more generally focused on whether inoculation should be performed at all. Later in the century, after inoculation had generally been accepted, medical practitioners argued over where inoculations should be performed – in hospital or at home. In each of these debates, mathematical arguments, similar in form to Nettleton's, were constructed, criticised, and refined. In this essay, I suggest that the mathematical approach indicated by merchant's logic and deployed in subsequent controversies over smallpox inoculation was a critical step to the development of medical statistics.[5]

Merchant's Logic and Medical Policy I:
To Inoculate or Not to Inoculate?

Nettleton applied merchant's logic – 'state the Account of Profitt and Loss to find on which side the Ballance Lyes' – by defining profit and loss in proportions that represented lives saved and lives lost to smallpox and to inoculation, that is, 1) the case fatality rate for natural smallpox; and 2) the case fatality rate for inoculated smallpox. The numerator in each of the ratios was the number of deaths due to either natural or inoculated smallpox. The denominator in the first instance was the total number of persons who had contracted smallpox and in the second, the total number of persons inoculated. For Nettleton, these proportions became measures of the hazards or odds of dying from natural and inoculated smallpox, and the profit clearly lay on the side of inoculation. Nettleton based his proportions on his own records and on information he gathered from neighbouring towns. He defined his populations solely by their experience with either natural or inoculated smallpox, a point his critics made, as I discuss below.

Nettleton recounted his experiences in a letter to Dr. William Whitaker (1696?-1743), a fellow Yorkshireman, who, while in London, forwarded the account to the Royal Society. Many members of the Society were interested in Nettleton's efforts, especially the secretary, the physician James Jurin (1684-1750), who eagerly sought him out regarding his experiences with inoculation. Nettleton's letters to Jurin contained the calculations and merchant's logic presented above – portions of which Jurin subsequently published in the *Philosophical Transactions.*[6]

Jurin, a successful London physician and Newtonian natural philosopher, extended Nettleton's merchant's logic in a series of pamphlets published annually from 1723 to 1727 and aptly entitled *An Account of the Success of Inoculating the Smallpox.*[7] Like Nettleton, Jurin provided proportions representing the case fatality rates of natural and inoculated smallpox, which demonstrated inoculation to be a beneficial practice. He based his ratios on figures drawn from reports by other physicians and surgeons throughout England and Wales of their experiences with natural and inoculated smallpox.[8] Specifically, Jurin collected accounts of inoculation, tallied the number of successes and failures (which he defined as deaths caused by inoculation), and constructed proportions expressing the hazard of dying from inoculation (roughly 1 in 91), much as Nettleton had done. Jurin also solicited and received surveys of natural smallpox mortality from individual physicians which indicated a 1 in 5 or 6 chance of dying once the disease had been contracted. Unlike Nettleton, Jurin augmented these figures for natural smallpox mortality by analysing the London bills of mortality.

The London bills of mortality listed the number of burials attributed to different diseases and casualties for each of London's parishes. Jurin's use of the bills indicates that he was familiar with John Graunt's *Natural and Political Observations made Upon the Bills of Mortality* (1662). In this pioneering work, Graunt calculated numerous proportions (e.g., ratios of the sexes or ratios of burials to christenings) and used these proportions to make a variety of observations on London's population. A careful and honest calculator, Graunt indicated a number of difficulties in using the bills, including problems of categorisation and under-reporting of certain groups (e.g., Dissenters) as well as of certain diseases. Despite these difficulties, he demonstrated that a range of useful and interesting conclusions could be drawn from a close study of the bills. Graunt referred to his calculations as being drawn from his 'shop-arithmetic' – a phrase reminiscent of Nettleton's merchant's logic.

Graunt's methods closely resembled double-entry book-keeping, a common commercial practice in which credits and debits were entered separately: one column tracked profits, and the other losses. Merchants assessed their financial status by comparing the balances in the two columns. As Philip Kreager has shown, book-keeping procedures from the late seventeenth century treated balances on a provisional and approximate basis, exactly as Graunt did with the bills of mortality. In Kreager's words: 'As long as the books (or bills) as a whole were well kept, isolated ratios or 'trial balances' could be accepted as accurate measures of profits and losses, which could then be numerically relevant to other 'accompts' and to the state of the people as a whole.'[9] This informal quality of accounting allowed Graunt, Nettleton, Jurin, and others to compare figures taken from very different populations.

When Jurin turned to the London bills of mortality to calculate the rate of natural smallpox mortality over a 45-year period, he encountered a number of problems that Nettleton's more direct counts had avoided. Most prominently, Jurin had to make assumptions about exposure to the disease. Accordingly, he reasoned that everyone in London was exposed to smallpox and concluded that those who survived infancy 'are all supposed to undergo that Disease sooner or later...'.[10] He also faced the problem of categorisation: smallpox was listed separately as a cause of death for the periods 1667–86 and 1701–22. During the intermediate years (1687–1700), smallpox and measles were recorded in the same category. For the two periods when smallpox was listed separately, Jurin constructed two tables which listed annual proportions representing smallpox mortality as a proportion of total mortality. These proportions fluctuated considerably from a high of 1 in 8 burials in 1674 and 1710 to a low of 1 in 149 burials in 1684; the average was 1 in 14 burials in and around London due to natural smallpox.[11]

Jurin's indebtedness to Graunt is further revealed by his decision to consider the effects of high infant mortality on his proportions. Graunt had recognised that certain diseases and casualties listed in the bills affected only infants and children, and he had calculated the proportion of burials attributed to these diseases, which revealed a high level of infant and child mortality.[12] Jurin followed a similar path. He specified the diseases affecting infants and children, such as 'overlaid' and 'Hooping Cough', and reasoned that these 'Articles in the Yearly Bills for the 22 years last past, amount as a Medium to 386 in each 1000, of the whole Number of Burials.' In other words, almost 40% of the burials were attributable to infant and child deaths.[13]

Jurin departed from Graunt in some respects, however. Graunt considered smallpox, swinepox, measles, and 'worms without Convulsions' as a single category, and had estimated that half of the total number of burials ascribed to these diseases were to children under six years old.[14] Jurin, on the other hand, assumed that these infants and young children died of other causes before being exposed to smallpox, a difference which illustrates the role of medical judgment in the assessment of the bills of mortality. 'It is notorious', Jurin commented, 'that great Numbers, especially of young Children, die of other Diseases, without ever having the Small Pox.'[15] Hence, Jurin subtracted the number of infant and child burials from the total number of burials and concluded that '*no more than between 7 and 8 can recover from that Distemper [smallpox] for one that dies of it*'.[16] Taking the high rate of infant mortality into account made the mortality figures for natural smallpox appear all the more grave.

Similarly to Graunt and Jurin, the physician John Arbuthnot (1667-1735) drew on the London bills to calculate mortality ratios for natural smallpox. Arbuthnot, a royal physician, was a keen advocate of mathematics and in 1701 had published *An Essay on the Usefulness of Mathematical Learning*. In his anonymous pamphlet, *Mr. Maitland's Account of Inoculating the Smallpox Vindicated* (1722), he presented a rougher set of calculations than did Jurin, but followed practically the same approach. First, Arbuthnot calculated the proportion of smallpox burials to total burials from the London bills of mortality as 1 in 12 for the twelve-year period from 1707–18. He then adjusted this proportion by subtracting infant mortality which he took to be roughly 25 per cent. He assumed that the overwhelming majority of infant deaths (8 in 9) were attributable to maladies other than smallpox, and recalculated the ratio of smallpox deaths to all other deaths as 1 in 10. Finally, he estimated the case fatality rate of inoculation as 1 in 100, however he provided no figures to support this estimation.[17]

Thus there were two basic methods developed by Nettleton,

Jurin, and Arbuthnot to evaluate the hazard or risk of inoculation: 1) to calculate the mortality of inoculated and natural smallpox based on actual accounts; and 2) to calculate smallpox mortality as a proportion of total mortality from the London bills of mortality. Each of these methods had its weaknesses as these physicians realised and as their critics pointed out. Jurin acknowledged the approximate nature of his calculations based on the bills of mortality (something, too, Graunt had assumed). Certainly Graunt's, Jurin's, and Arbuthnot's assessment of infant mortality from the bills reflected this approximate quality. Their manipulation of the London bills also shows that the Bills could not simply be read; they had to be interpreted.

Jurin, however, sought something more than an approximation and recommended that a 'careful Person' carry out a house-to-house survey to discover how many contracted smallpox and of those how many died. This method, Jurin argued, 'would enable us to come at a nearer and still more certain Computation of the Proportion between those that recover, and those that die of the Small Pox'.[18] But even this approach did not answer all the critics: relying on tallies of who had contracted smallpox and who had been inoculated ignored the fact that these two populations were often in quite dissimilar circumstances, both bodily and financially.[19]

The numerical arguments developed by Nettleton, Jurin, and Arbuthnot during the debates over smallpox inoculation in the 1720s became central to determinations of medical practice and policy. Regardless of the particular faults of each type of calculation, a rational individual following merchant's logic (that is, a commercially-minded person) could compare the two ratios and easily decide on which side the profit lay. For all three men, the hazard of dying from natural smallpox was much greater than the hazard of dying from inoculation. By comparing the mortality ratios, Jurin asserted, 'the Publick may be enabled to form a Judgment, whether or not the Practice of Inoculation tends to the Preservation of Mankind, by lessening the Danger to which they are otherwise liable'.[20] Jurin agreed with Nettleton's aim to evaluate the benefit of inoculation for the public, which Jurin defined as 'the preservation of Mankind'. In this sense, profit once again was defined in terms of lives saved. But it is important to emphasise that Jurin erased references to merchants' practices. Instead he appealed to the disinterested qualities of numerical arguments. 'I heartily wish, that, without Passion, Prejudice, or private Views', he concluded, inoculation 'may be fairly and maturely examin'd. In order to which ... the following Extracts and computations concerning the comparative Danger of the inoculated and Natural Small Pox may be of use....'[21]

Arbuthnot, too, did not refer to merchant's logic when he reflected on the meaning of his calculations, although the language of profits and losses clearly comes across.

> A Practice which brings the Mortality of the Small Pox from one in ten to one in a hundred, it if obtain'd universally would save to the City of London at least 1500 People yearly; and the same Odds wou'd be a sufficient prudential Motive to any private Person to proceed upon, abstracting from the more occult and abstruse Causes which seem to favour this operation. It is a self evident proposition, that a Person who receives the Infection by Inoculation, has a much fairer Chance for his life, than he who takes it the Natural Way...[22]

Arbuthnot combined the language of political arithmetic with the language of individual risk. His figures supported inoculation first by revealing the advantages to the state (a larger population) and second by commenting on how odds should motivate rational behaviour, much like merchant's logic. Individual profit (self-interest) and public profit (common benefit or commonwealth) went hand in hand. The form of Jurin's and Arbuthnot's arguments shared many characteristics of Graunt's shop-arithmetic and Nettleton's merchant's logic, although neither Jurin nor Arbuthnot referred to their mathematical approaches as commercial in origin. The reason for this was no doubt social. As prominent London physicians and members of the Royal Society and the Royal College of Physicians, Jurin and Arbuthnot avoided mention of merchants' practices and preferred instead to couch their arguments in terms of the mathematics that one would find at a meeting of gentlemanly natural philosophers.

Merchant's Logic and Medical Policy II: inoculate at home or in hospital?

By 1750, inoculation had become generally accepted in England, in part due to the numerical arguments and in part due to its adoption by the Royal Family and members of the aristocracy. This at least was the assessment presented by the physician James MacKenzie in the third edition of his popular *History of Health* (1760). Citing a Dr. Davies of Bath, Mackenzie wrote

> That inoculation was not stifled in the bud by the prevailing passions and prejudices of mankind, we owe chiefly to two

favourable circumstances, *viz.* to the countenance it received from the Royal Family, and to the abilities and integrity of Dr. Jurin, who undertook the office of candid historian, putting that practice to the fair test of experience.[23]

By mid-century, the wealthy had embraced the practice and their children were routinely inoculated at home with all the possible care physicians and surgeons could furnish.

Those of less means had fewer choices. In 1746, the Smallpox Hospital was established in London as a charity to inoculate the poor and to nurse those who had contracted smallpox. But one institution alone could do little to aid London's burgeoning poor population. In other parts of the country, many individual surgeons and physicians established private inoculation houses during the second half of the eighteenth century.[24] For a fee, a person could reside in one of these houses for the duration of the illness caused by inoculation. The fear of contagion, however, forced many of these private houses to relocate or close.[25] Given the inadequacies of these few institutions and the widespread acceptance of inoculation as a beneficial practice, the issue of inoculating the poor gained urgency, especially during smallpox epidemics.[26] It became, along with other charitable causes such as prison reform and slavery abolition, a favourite objective of many prominent dissenting physicians, including the Quaker John Coakley Lettsom and Thomas Dimsdale (born a Quaker), who took the lead in promoting inoculation during the second half of the eighteenth century.[27]

While consensus reigned in regards to the advantages of inoculating the poor, dispute and debate were the rule in discussions about where to inoculate individuals. According to one critic, inoculation hospitals fell short on four grounds. First, they could admit only a limited number of poor each year. Second, they did not allow the cold air treatment for smallpox advocated by Thomas Sydenham. Third, the poor were fearful of putting themselves in the care of nurses rather than of family; and finally, the air was impure in hospitals. Thus, this critic continued, 'To obviate these objections, and to render the practice of Inoculation more general; it has been thought expedient to establish a Dispensary for Inoculating the Poor.'[28]

Many echoed these sentiments during the last decades of the eighteenth century. In 1775, for example, the philanthropic 'Society for the Inoculation of the Poor', whose members included the physicians John Watkinson and John Coakley Lettsom, was founded in London to promote the inoculation of the poor in their homes.[29] Such a plan would decrease the expense of the practice and extend its benefits to a far greater proportion of the population. In fact, in some rural towns where smallpox was not endemic, general inoculations of the entire population had been carried out in the face of an imminent smallpox epidemic.[30] While general inoculations were feasible for villages and small communities, they could not be easily carried out in large cities such as London, Manchester or Liverpool. Public dispensaries or inoculations at home were two solutions to delivering inoculation to a larger segment of the urban population, but efforts to establish dispensaries met with resistance because of the belief that inoculated smallpox was highly contagious and thus could trigger an epidemic; therefore, critics argued, inoculation should be performed in hospital under professional supervision.

The most prominent advocate of inoculation hospitals was Thomas Dimsdale, a physician who had received fame, title, and fortune (£10,000) for inoculating the Empress of Russia in 1768. Firmly convinced that inoculating the urban poor in their homes would spread smallpox, he instead proposed a plan for inoculation hospitals – such as the London Smallpox Hospital – that would provide adequate supervision of both the physicians and the poor undergoing inoculation. Dimsdale's 1776 pamphlet, *Thoughts on General and Partial Inoculations*, addressed to Parliament, argued that inoculation should be regulated 'for the mischief arising from the practice of inoculation by the illiterate and ignorant is beyond conception'.[31] Dimsdale's private practice of inoculating wealthy patients, however, made his opinion of public inoculations of the urban poor vulnerable to attack: 'though he demonstrates himself no friend to inoculation of the poor, [he] seems to have little objection to inoculation of the rich: perhaps this is rather too lucrative a branch of his own business to be readily given up', charged an anonymous pamphleteer.[32]

In the debate over where to inoculate the urban poor, medical men on both sides of the issue turned to quantitative arguments based on figures culled from the London bills of mortality in order to assess the effects of inoculation on smallpox mortality and thus to adduce the risks of contagion from inoculated smallpox. If inoculated smallpox did indeed provoke epidemics, as one version of the argument went, general smallpox mortality would have increased after the introduction of the practice in London in the 1720s. If such an increase could be documented, then it would provide evidence against the establishment of dispensaries to inoculate London's poor.

Alternatively, others argued that an increase in smallpox mortality reflected the failure to practice inoculation, and that through the establishment of dispensaries a large number of individuals could be inoculated, hence lowering the rate of smallpox mortality. Both arguments were based on the earlier quantitative work on the hazards of inoculation and in their form followed the merchant's logic: that is, they summed the costs and benefits to assess on which side profit lay. The relationship between individual risk and common good varied, however; private and public interest did not always coincide. A few examples will illustrate these differences.

The writer of the tract cited above which outlined the liabilities of smallpox hospitals employed a political arithmetical argument much like Arbuthnot's of the 1720s. The anonymous author presented the total number of London inhabitants who had perished from smallpox during the last 50 years (a figure taken directly from the London bills of mortality). This was the simplest use of the Bills. He then argued that if these individuals had been inoculated, 'the number of lives which would have been thereby redeemed, together with the probable encrease from them, must have made a very considerable addition to the strength of the state.' These population considerations made it a moral and political duty to inoculate, as the opening paragraph of the pamphlet made explicit: 'As the strength of a nation is in some measure proportionate to the number of its inhabitants, every attempt to encrease population, by preserving life, has a just claim to the regard both of Patriotism and Humanity.'[33] Since inoculation hospitals were inadequate according to this author and private benefit and public welfare went hand in hand, London should have more dispensaries to inoculate the poor.

John Watkinson, one of the members of the Society for the Inoculation of the Poor, challenged this approach of simply presenting the total number of deaths attributed to smallpox – an approach which did not take into account the increase in London's population. Since London's population was continually fluctuating, Watkinson argued, 'no certain conclusion can possibly be drawn, with respect to the increase or decrease of the mortality of the small-pox, from the *absolute* number of deaths by that disease in one period, compared with the absolute number of deaths by the same disease in another period.'[34] In fact, absolute numbers were a problem for all those who worked with the bills of mortality. As many observers noted, the total number of annual deaths presented in the bills had remained roughly the same throughout the century. 'The bills for the five years 1701-1705, amounted to 105,453, those for the five years 1710-1714, to 113,277, and those for the five years 1771-1775, only to 110,887', one contributor remarked. 'Yet that there must have been a very great addition to the numbers of London within the present century will be allowed by every thinking man who finds no visible diminution of population with such prodigious augmentation of building.' This author accounted for the discrepancy by pointing to more efficacious medicine, a greater salubrity of air, and the tendency of individuals to go to the countryside to die.[35]

To avoid the problems raised by simply taking the absolute numbers listed in the bills, Watkinson advocated the method found in the writings of Richard Price, known best for his work on annuities. Followers of Price, according to Watkinson, 'endeavoured to trace the variations in the mortality of this distemper [smallpox], not from the *absolute*, but the *relative* number of its victims, that is, from the proportion which they bore to those of all the other diseases at one time, compared with the proportions which they bore them at another'.[36] This was precisely the method developed by Jurin and Arbuthnot in the 1720s. Accordingly, Watkinson constructed a table indicating the proportions of 'the mean annual number of deaths by the smallpox, compared with the mean annual number of deaths by all the other diseases.'[37]

Year	Ratio of smallpox to other deaths
1714–1720	1 to 11
1721–1727	1 to 11
1728–1734	1 to 12
1735–1741	1 to 13
1742–1748	1 to 13
1749–1755	1 to 11
1756–1762	1 to 9

Before inoculation, roughly 1 in 11 burials was attributed to smallpox. After inoculation, the proportion varied from 1 in 9 to 1 in 13 burials. Watkinson asked:

whether the number of deaths by the small-pox has risen and fallen, in proportion as inoculation has been more or less practised. If this should be the case, there will be some reason for imputing that variation to inoculation. But if on the contrary it should appear, that the one has not corresponded to the other, it will be evident, that the increase of mortality, and the practice of inoculation are not connected together as cause and effect.[38]

His proportions showed that the rate of smallpox mortality had remained roughly the same before and after inoculation, thus he concluded that there was no positive correlation between the practice of inoculation and the increase in smallpox mortality, and hence no sound argument against dispensaries for inoculating the poor.[39] For Watkinson, the liabilities of dispensaries were outweighed by the advantages of extending inoculation to the poor, a point he made by invoking a utilitarian version of merchant's logic: the 'sum of the *good* produced by Inoculation is far greater than that of the *evil*'.[40]

Dimsdale drew precisely the opposite conclusions from similar calculations and contended that smallpox was 'equally fatal' in London despite inoculation. In order to prove his point, Dimsdale extended Jurin's table of smallpox mortality for 34 years (1734 - 67 inclusive) taken from the bills of mortality. Like Jurin, Dimsdale deducted the number of burials attributed to infants and children under two years of age. He showed that smallpox mortality remained constant in London (1 in 8) since inoculation had been introduced during the 1720s, and concluded that the practice had little effect on general smallpox mortality.[41] For him, public welfare and private benefit would go hand in hand only if inoculation were performed in hospitals; this would protect the general population from the risks of smallpox infection and greater mortality.

An anonymous pamphlet entitled *Considerations on the Propriety of a Plan for Inoculating the Poor of London at their own Habitations* (1779) presented a method similar to Watkinson's but with very different results. The author compared the proportion of deaths due to smallpox to total deaths for 42 years preceding the introduction of inoculation to the 42 years following its introduction. The figures for the first 42-year period (72 of 1000 or 1 in 14) were taken from Jurin's calculations. The figures for the second 42-year period, which the pamphleteer calculated himself, displayed a range from 77 of 1000 or 1 in 13 to 105 of 1000 or 1 in 9 1/2. 'The result of this comparison is', the author claimed, 'that the Small Pox has increased very considerably in its fatality during the latter period', precisely because of inoculation.[42] 'The conclusion which presents itself to a candid inquirer', he asserted, 'is that the benefits derived to individuals have been more than balanced by the evils which have arisen from diffusing the contagion.'[43] This was a clear statement of merchant's logic and indicated that the public's interest was not being served by private inoculation, or in other words inoculation at home through a dispensary. Profit was now defined solely in terms of public welfare rather than individual benefit; the two no longer coincided as they had in the eyes of Nettleton, Jurin, and Arbuthnot.

In all of these arguments, the authors were hampered by a lack of reliable information about the actual practice of inoculation in London; attempts to infer the extent of inoculation from smallpox mortality figures could be used to support quite opposite positions. Numerical arguments incorporated various forms of merchant's logic, most often balancing profit and loss in terms of public good (measured by gross smallpox mortality or the proportion of smallpox mortality to total mortality) and private benefit (measured by the risks of dying from inoculation). The only exception was Thomas Dimsdale. He had no truck with this argument, and in fact rejected the underlying proposition of merchant's logic: 'Can a man be so unfeeling as to reason coolly on the sum of the good and evil produced, where the lives of fellow-mortals, equally precious to the poor as to the rich, are the objects?'[44] Dimsdale espoused a Romantic characterisation of Enlightenment numerical arguments as 'unfeeling' and indicative of 'reasoning coolly'. Numbers were persuasive precisely because they were impersonal, but, by the same measure, they were also insensitive because they valued the welfare of the population over the welfare of the individual.

Conclusion

In this essay, I have explored the place of merchant's logic in the formulation and acceptance of numerical arguments in two of the many debates surrounding smallpox inoculation. How successful was merchant's logic? Very few individuals completely dismissed numerical arguments as irrelevant to medicine, such that by the end of the eighteenth century, even those opposed to the practice of inoculation in certain circumstances justified their position on the basis of numerical arguments. Although physicians were unlikely to refer to commercial or merchant practices explicitly in their writings, the actual form of their arguments (a sort of rough cost-benefit analysis) as well as their choice of language reflected contemporary accounting practices. Physicians found these types of arguments persuasive, which might in part be due to the larger cultural changes occurring in Britain. The introduction and acceptance of numerical methods into British medicine can be treated as part of the emerging commercial and consumer culture of the period.[45]

Merchant's logic entered eighteenth-century British medicine in less methodologically explicit ways as well. Recently historians have examined the role of the state (for example, of the Excise Office) in introducing precise measurement and recording techniques into traditional craft practices.[46] Theodore Porter has labelled this process the 'accounting ideal' of science and discussed how practical and commercial needs increased the use of quantification and precise measurements.[47] I would like to suggest that a similar process occurred in medicine. In particular, the growth of charity hospitals and dispensaries, institutions financially beholden to their subscribers, encouraged the development of more accurate accounting techniques, which, like Nettleton's merchant's logic, brought forms of commercial rationality into medicine. The Smallpox Hospital, for example, published several reports to inform potential and actual subscribers about the activities of the hospital. The Governors presented a balance of expenses, including an account of the number of patients. From 26 January 1746 to 31 December 1752, 1352 patients were treated for natural smallpox of whom 1033 were cured. During the same period, 131 individuals were inoculated of whom 2 died.[48] A subsequent report published two years later presented additional figures on the efficacy of the practice. From 31 December 1751 to 31 December 1755, 593 persons were inoculated, and 'that out of this large number of 593, only *one* has died; while this terrible Distemper taken by the common, unperceived Infection (usually called the *Natural* way) destroys, *at least,* one in Seven (perhaps in a greater Proportion) of those who are seized with it.' Here the Governors made much the same argument that Nettleton and Jurin had made, only they based their conclusions on an account of their own patients. In seeking additional benefactors, the Governors displayed these figures. They also included a description of how patients were inoculated in the hospital, and indicated the care taken at the hospital.[49] Donating to the Smallpox Hospital therefore could be judged a good investment on many counts.

The example of the Smallpox Hospital is straightforward in its connection between fiscal needs and medical practice, and it illustrates how pressures of public justification (accountability) encouraged quantitative accounts of patients. More broadly, smallpox inoculation served as a lightning-rod for the development of numerical, commercial arguments in eighteenth-century British medicine. It was a specific medical practice whose benefits and risks (both private and public) could be assessed quantitatively. This type of rationale is now common – indeed essential – to establishing new therapies, and it had its roots in eighteenth century debates over smallpox inoculation.

Notes

1. For historical accounts of inoculation in England see: Genevieve Miller, *The Adoption of Inoculation for Smallpox in England and France* (Philadelphia: University of Pennsylvania Press, 1957); and Peter Razzell, *The Conquest of Smallpox: The Impact of Inoculation on Smallpox Mortality in Eighteenth Century Britain* (Sussex: Caliban Books, 1977); J.R. Smith, *The Speckled Monster: Smallpox in England, 1670-1970, with particular reference to Essex* (Chelmsford: Essex Record Office, 1987).

2. Thomas Nettleton to James Jurin, 16 December 1722 in *The Correspondence of James Jurin (1684-1750)*, Andrea Rusnock (ed.), (Amsterdam and Atlanta: Rodopi Press, 1996), 117–120.

3. Thomas Nettleton to James Jurin, 24 January 1723, in *ibid.*, 125–127.

4. On the politics of inoculation see Adrian Wilson, 'The politics of medical improvement in early Hanoverian London', in Andrew Cunningham and Roger French (eds), *The Medical Enlightenment of the Eighteenth Century* (Cambridge: Cambridge University Press, 1990), 4–39; and Francis M. Lobo, 'John Haygarth, Smallpox and Religious Dissent in Eighteenth-century England', *ibid.*, 217–253.

5. For an overview of medical statistics in England during the eighteenth century see Major Greenwood, *Medical Statistics from Graunt to Farr* (Cambridge: Cambridge University Press, 1948). More recently, Ulrich Troehler has focused on the use of numerical methods by English physicians and surgeons during the latter half of the eighteenth century. See Ulrich Troehler, 'Quantification in British Medicine and Surgery 1750-1830, with Special Reference to its Introduction into Therapeutics', Ph.D. Dissertation, University of London, 1978; *idem*, '"To Improve the Evidence of Medicine": Arithmetic Observation in Clinical Medicine in the 18th and Early 19th Centuries', *History and Philosophy of the Life Sciences Supplement* x (1988), 31–40. For the classic statement on the origin of medical statistics in Parisian hospital medicine see Erwin Ackerknecht, *Medicine at the Paris Hospital 1794-1848* (Baltimore: Johns Hopkins University Press, 1967).

6. Thomas Nettleton, 'A Letter form Dr. Nettleton', *Philosophical Transactions* 32(1722), 51; Nettleton, 'Part of a Letter from Dr.

Nettleton', *Philosophical Transactions* 32(1722), 209–212.

7. See James Jurin: 'A Letter to the Learned Caleb Cotesworth, MD,
    FRS, of the College of Physicians, and Physician to St. Thomas's
    Hospital, Containing A Comparison between the Mortality of the
    Natural Small Pox, and that given by Inoculation', *Philosophical
    Transactions* 1723, 32: 213–24, and published separately as a
    pamphlet with additions, *A Letter to the Learned Caleb Cotesworth...
    Which is Subjoined an Account of the Success of Inoculation in New-
    England; As Likewise an Extract from Several Letters concerning a Like
    Method of Communicating the Small-Pox, That Has Been Used Time
    Out of Mind in South Wales* (London, 1723); *An Account of the
    Success of Inoculating the Small Pox in Great Britain with a
    Comparison Between the Miscarriages in that Practice, and the
    Mortality of the Natural Small Pox* (London, 1724); *An Account of the
    Success of Inoculating the Small Pox for the Year 1724* (London, 1725);
    *An Account of the Success of Inoculating the Small Pox for the Year
    1725* (London, 1726); *An Account of the Success of Inoculating the
    Small Pox for the Year 1726* (London 1727).

8. For an account of Jurin's project see Andrea Rusnock, 'The Weight
    of Evidence and the Burden of Authority: Case Histories, Medical
    Statistics and Smallpox Inoculation', *Medicine in the Enlightenment*,
    Roy Porter (ed.), (Amsterdam and Atlanta: Rodopi Press, 1995),
    289–315.

9. Philip Kreager, 'New Light on Graunt', *Population Studies* 42 (1988),
    129–40: 136.

10. Jurin, *op. cit.* (note 7), 221.

11. *Ibid.*, 216–18.

12. John Graunt, *Natural and Political Observations Made Upon the Bills
    of Mortality*, 5th edn,[1676], in Charles Henry Hull (ed.), *The
    Economic Writings of Sir William Petty* (Cambridge: Cambridge
    University Press, 1899), 315–431, 349, 359, and 362–3.
    Subsequent citations to Graunt refer to this edition.

13. Jurin, *op. cit.* (note 7), 220.

14. Graunt, *op. cit.* (note 12), 349.

15. Jurin, *op. cit.* (note 7), 219. By the end of the eighteenth century,
    this judgement had been reversed. More precise bills of mortality
    which included age of death indicated that smallpox was most
    deadly for infants and children from age 6 months to 3 years. See
    Thomas Percival, 'Essay II. on the Small-Pox and Measles', *London
    Medical Observations and Inquiries*, vol. V (1789), 270; reprinted in
    Population and Disease in Early Industrial England, intro. B.
    Benjamin (Gregg International Publishers Limited, 1973).

16. Jurin, *op. cit.* (note 7), 221.

17. [John Arbuthnot], *Mr. Maitland's Account of Inoculating the Smallpox Vindicated, From Dr. Wagstaffe's Misrepresentations of that Practice, with some Remarks on Mr. Massey's Sermon* (London, 1722), 18–20.

18. Jurin, *op. cit.* (note 7), 222.

19. See, for example, Isaac Massey, *A Short and Plain Account of Inoculation*, 2nd edn (London, 1723), 2–3.

20. Jurin, *op. cit.* (note 7), 215–6.

21. *Ibid.*, 214.

22. *Maitland's Account … Vindicated, op. cit.* (note 17), 25.

23. James Mackenzie, *The History of Health, and the Art of Preserving It, Third Edition, to which is added, a short and clear Account of the Commencement, Progress, Utility, and proper Management of Inoculating the Small Pox, as a valuable Branch of the Prophylaxis* (Edinburgh: William Gordon, 1760), 430.

24. See Miller, *op. cit.* (note 1), 146–56.

25. *Ibid.*, 165–8.

26. *Ibid.*, 146.

27. Robert Kilpatrick, '"Living in the light": dispensaries, philanthropy and medical reform in late-eighteenth-century London', in Andrew Cunningham and Roger French (eds), *The Medical Enlightenment of the Eighteenth Century* (Cambridge: Cambridge University Press, 1990), 254–80.

28. *Plan of a Dispensary for Inoculating the Poor*, n.p., n.d.

29. See James Johnston Abraham, *Lettsom - His Life, Times, Friends and Descendants* (London: William Heinemann, 1933), 196–7.

30. Miller, *op. cit.* (note 1), 155.

31. Thomas Dimsdale, *Thoughts on General and Partial Inoculations* (London: William Richardson, 1776), 9.

32. Anonymous, *A Letter to J.C. Lettsom, M.D., FRS, SAS &c Occasioned by Baron Dimsdale's Remarks on Dr. Lettsom's Letter to Sir Robert Barker, and G. Stacpoole, esq. upon General Inoculation* (London: J. Murray, 1779), 32.

33. *Plan of a Dispensary for Inoculating the Poor*, n.p., n.d.

34. John Watkinson, *An Examination of a Charge Brought Against Inoculation, by DeHaen, Rast, Dimsdale, and other Writers* (London: J. Johnson, 1778), 4.

35. Anonymous, *A Letter to J.C. Lettsom, M.D.*, 9–10.

36. Watkinson, *op. cit.* (note 34), 5.

37. *Ibid.*, 27.

38. *Ibid.*, 26–7.

39. Watkinson's logic was somewhat convoluted on this point: 'That the

prevalence of inoculation, and the increased mortality of the
smallpox, have in no point coincided, I do not mean to insinuate.
According to the laws of chance, this must sometimes have
happened. But I contend, that the great irregularity of their
coincidence may be considered as a fresh proof, that the one, is not
the cause of the other.' *Ibid.*, 29.

40. Cited in Thomas Dimsdale, *Observations on the Introduction to the Plan of the Dispensary for General Inoculation* (London, 1778), 61.

41. Thomas Dimsdale, *Thoughts on General and Partial Inoculations* (London: William Richardson, 1776), 13.

42. *Considérations on the Propriety of a Plan for Inoculating the Poor of London at their own Habitations* (London, 1779), 5.

43. *Ibid.*, 6.

44. Thomas Dimsdale, *Observations on the Introduction of the Plan of the Dispensary for General Inoculation* (London, 1778), 117–118.

45. Neil McKendrick, John Brewer, and J.H. Plumb, *The Birth of a Consumer Society* (London: Hutchinson & Co., 1982).

46. John Brewer, *The Sinews of Power* (NY: Alfred Knopf, 1988), Ch. 8, 'The Politics of Information'; Theodore Porter, *Trust in Numbers: The Pursuit of Objectivity in Science and Public Life* (Princeton: Princeton University Press, 1995), 50–1.

47. Theodore Porter, 'Quantification and the Accounting Ideal in Science', *Social Studies of Science* 22(1992), 633–52.

48. *An Account of the Rise, Progress and State of the Hospital, for relieving poor People afflicted with the Small Pox, and for Inoculation*, n.p., n.d. [1754].

49. *A Representation from the Governors of the Hospital for the Small-Pox and for Inoculation*, n.p., n.d. [1756].

3

The Annual Report of the Registrar General, 1839–1920:
A Textual History[1]

Edward Higgs

The General Register Office and the history of statistics

This paper is not strictly about the use of statistics in medical research. Rather, it attempts to reconstruct the factors influencing the publishing history of that central text of Victorian and Edwardian statistical medicine, the *Annual Report of the Registrar General*. This was the main publishing venture of the General Register Office (GRO). Established in 1837, this office was responsible for supervising the secular system for registering births, marriages and deaths set up in England and Wales under the provisions of the 1836 Registration and Marriage Acts. The civil registration system replaced the former arrangements for the registration of baptisms, marriages and burials via the clergy of the Church of England. The GRO maintained a central 'database' of copies of the certificates of registration of vital events issued by local registrars, from which it produced weekly, quarterly, annual and decennial reports on medical and demographic trends. Although the greatest range of material was provided at the national level, important data were published down to the level of individual named districts. A key element of this process was the analysis of cause of death data supplied on death certificates, which helped underpin both advances in medical science and the Victorian public health movement. The recording of the incidence of death from certain causes enabled doctors to study the geographical and temporal patterns of disease, whilst information on variations in the number of deaths per thousand in defined administrative units highlighted the need for local sanitary reform.[2] From 1841 the GRO was also responsible for the taking of the decennial census.[3]

The approach employed here, an analysis of the publishing history of a statistical text, is in marked contrast to the recent historiography of the development of statistics as a branch of mathematical logic based on concepts of probability and error.[4] But any attempt to analyse the statistical work of the GRO in the Victorian period along these lines would be comparatively fruitless. In truth, the GRO's mathematical skills were limited, on the whole, to the calculation of life tables, and to the comparison of raw aggregates and simple ratios. The stock in trade of William Farr, the GRO's superintendent of statistics from 1839 to 1879, was the table showing local variations in the rate of deaths per thousand, rather than the use of equations or probabilities. For Farr 'statistics' was not strictly a branch of mathematics but a much broader 'science of States – the science of men living in political communities...'.[5] This meant the comparison of nations rather than the study of normal distributions. Farr's ideal for the statistical project was the establishment of a common framework for national statistics to allow international comparisons.[6]

This overarching concept of statistics was undermined in the late Victorian and Edwardian period by the emergence of modern mathematical statistics from the work of men such as Francis Galton and Karl Pearson.[7] Eugenicists such as Galton were not concerned with reducing national differences to averages, but in measuring the differences which existed between individual human beings. Farr, following the great Belgian statist Adolphe Quetelet, sought to create a picture of the social average, whilst Galton and Pearson wished to show the differences over time in the characteristics of differing groups with diverse genetic endowments.[8] This led the latter to develop the modern statistical methods for measuring dispersion, distribution and probabilities within data. This contrast can be seen in the clash between Farr and Galton over the lack of mathematical rigour in the work of the statistical section of the British Association for the Advancement of Science. For example, under Farr's direction the Association's Anthropometric Committee used simple relationships such as the comparison of mean values, whilst under Galton its work included the use of probability theory, normal distributions, and the quartile and decile as well as the mean. By the time of his death (1883), Farr's grandiose concept of statistics was already being discredited.[9]

The changing form and content of the Annual Report: 1839–1920

Despite the extensive use made of the GRO's reports by medical and demographic historians, and the general high esteem in which they are held, there has been little attempt to examine their changing form and structure, or the history of their production.[10] In the absence of a collected series of these publications, and adequate indexes to them, this scholarly omission is understandable. However, the absence of an overall appreciation of the form and content of the GRO's publishing endeavours disguises some of the important features of the Office's development, and leads to confusion. The first task here will be, therefore, to sketch out the gross features of this textual history from 1839 to the early-1920s.

As noted above, the centre-piece of the GRO's publishing endeavours was the *Annual Report of the Registrar General,* which discussed the registration, demographic and medical data abstracted for a single twelve-month period. The report might appear up to 40 months after the year upon which it commented, although an interval of a year was more usual. As can be seen from Figure 1, these delays were greatest in the early decades of the GRO's existence but nearly always grew in the first half of each decade, before declining in the second. This pattern is probably explained by the large amounts of extra work which the planning, taking and reporting of the census created for the Office every ten years. The 1841 census was, of course, the first the GRO organised, and that of 1851 was in many ways its most ambitious,[11] and this may explain, in part, the extreme delays in producing the *Annual Reports* in these decades. The GRO attempted to get round this problem by producing a shorter abstract which was laid before parliament, and publishing the full report with explanatory text separately at a later date. Thus, a general abstract for 1848 had been laid before Parliament in 1850,[12] but the full report was not completed until December 1851, and not published by the Stationery Office until 1852.[13] This means that, confusingly, the *Annual Reports* found amongst the published *Parliamentary Papers* are not necessarily the full texts.[14]

The text of the *Annual Report* was usually in two parts – the Registrar General's own report proper, and the 'Letter to the Registrar General' under the signature of the superintendent of statistics, each with appended tables. The former was usually a broad brush reflection on trends in vital events, with digressions on such matters as the ability of people to sign the marriage register, the relationship between marriage rates and the economy, and the effect of the weather on death rates. For much of the 1850s and 1860s this also included a summary of the quarterly reports on mortality in the various registration districts. The superintendent of statistic's 'Letter' was a less constant feature of the *Annual Report,* as can be seen from Figure 2.[15] In many years the Registrar General's own report was larger, and even during Farr's period of office the Letter might not appear at all.[16] As Simon Szreter notes, the 'Letter' signed by the statistical superintendent disappeared in the *Report* for 1879, only returning in that for 1901.[17] However, during these years the content of the 'Letter' was in fact incorporated into the Registrar General's own report under the heading 'Registered Causes of Death'. The *Reports* of the 1880s and 1890s were, on the whole, slighter documents than those which preceded and followed them. With the *Annual Report* for 1901 the division between the Registrar General's report and the Letter reasserted itself.[18] From the *Annual Report* for 1909 onwards, however, the Registrar General's own signed report became a mere few pages of introduction to the superintendent's Letter, now renamed the 'Review of Vital Statistics'.[19] The *Annual Report* for 1920 was in fact an unsigned version of the superintendent of statistic's 'Review'.[20] The following year this anonymous format continued but the whole was now retitled *The Registrar General's Statistical Review for 1921*.[21] The *Statistical Review*, unlike its predecessor, was no longer placed before parliament as a parliamentary paper.

The history of the *Annual Report* can thus be divided into four distinct periods: (i) the joint publication of reports by the Registrar Generals and Farr, covering the period 1839 to 1879; (ii) the last twenty years of the Victorian period, which saw the absorption of the Letter into the Registrar General's own report, coupled with a general decline in the GRO's output;[22] (iii) the rebirth of the separate superintendent of statistics' letter, with an expansion of publishing activity in the *Reports* from 1902 to 1909, and the absorption of the Registrar General's contribution into that of his statistical subordinate. This development terminated (iv) with the imposition of anonymity, and a new title in the 1920s. Such a pattern of expansion, retrenchment, revival and sudden termination in the history of the *Annual Report* reflects distinct phases in the administrative and political history of the GRO, which will be explored in the rest of this paper.[23]

The years of expansion, 1839 to 1879

In a sense, it is not the irregularity of the appearance of Farr's Letter in the early *Annual Reports* which needs to be explained but its gradual evolution into a permanent feature of the publication. After all, the GRO had not originally been established to publish statistical data, rather its purpose had been to underpin property rights via the recording of lines of descent.[24] The 1836 Registration Act only empowered the Registrar General to 'send once in every year to one of the principal secretaries of state a general abstract of the numbers of births, deaths, and marriages registered during the foregoing year, in such form as the said secretary from time to time shall require.'[25] In the first *Annual Report*, Farr's 'Letter' was only one of 16 appendices.[26] The origins of the GRO's statistical functions appear to have lain as much, if not more, in the interests of Edwin Chadwick and the Treasury in providing actuarial data for friendly societies, than in the needs of the medical profession.[27]

The gradual consolidation of the GRO's medical statistical functions depended to a considerable extent on the success of the Office in building up its Statistical Department. Thus, the staffing of this section of the GRO increased from four to 16 in the period 1840 to 1866.[28] Such an expansion in staff resources depended upon getting the support of the Treasury for increased expenditure. This was achieved, in part, through the success of William Farr's use of statistical data as a propaganda weapon on behalf of the public health movement. As Simon Szreter has stressed, Farr used the differences in the published rates of deaths per thousand in the various registration districts to highlight local sanitary failings. Thus, the 1848 Public Health Act[29] contained a provision that local authorities could be compelled to establish boards of health to implement local sanitary reform if their annual mortality rates were found to be above 23 per thousand, the national average at the time as measured by the GRO. In the course of the 1850s Farr developed the concept of the 'healthy districts'' mortality experience, based originally on a set of 63 registration districts, whose crude death rate was below 17 per thousand. This was then advocated as the desirable national standard, and deaths in excess of this were designated as preventable. The GRO shamed local authorities into sanitary reforms by publishing calculations indicating that tens of thousands of deaths in various cities would never have occurred if only the sanitary conditions of these districts approximated to those of the 'healthy districts'.[30] This role gave the GRO leverage with the Treasury when seeking resources.

But the expansion of the provision of medical data in the GRO also reflected demands from within Whitehall, which the Office turned to account in its dealings with the Treasury. As soon as the GRO began to publish data it came to be seen as a resource upon which others could draw. As early as March 1840, for example, Thomas Lister, the first Registrar General, was writing to the Treasury for provision for overtime working to handle a request from Parliament for a return of the number of people who died of smallpox in 1839.[31] Similarly, at the beginning of 1846, the Registrar General wrote to the Treasury indicating that he had been asked by the Home

Secretary to improve the range of mortality statistics published in the *Annual Report,* which would necessitate the addition of five extra staff to Farr's department. This was the result of an approach made to the Home Office by the British Association for the Advancement of Science.[32]

The expanded resources of the Statistical Department were to be fully stretched by the demands placed upon it by the General Board of Health. The Board, set up under the 1848 Public Health Act, and with Edwin Chadwick as its secretary, appears to have regarded the GRO as a limitless resource upon which it could draw. As already noted, under the Act local boards of health were to be set up if the death rate rose above 23 per 1,000 over the previous seven years. As a result, the Board bombarded the GRO with requests for information on general death rates for specific towns and districts, as well as for numerous ad hoc returns on specific diseases.[33] Indeed, so voracious was the Board for information that it had its own staff based at the GRO to work upon the registration data.[34]

The winding up of the General Board of Health in 1858 did not result in any diminution of demands for medical data by government departments. Indeed, John Simon, the medical officer of health at the Privy Council Office from 1858, proved an even more avid consumer of data. From this position Simon took up the running as the dynamic centre of public health administration in central government. This had an almost immediate impact on the work of the GRO. Simon obtained permission from the GRO to have one of his own clerks work through the GRO's mortality data to produce figures for deaths by various causes broken down by districts.[35] The resulting *Papers Relating to the Sanitary State of the People of England* went beyond the GRO's practice of only publishing total mortality rates.[36] Similarly, Simon arranged for the GRO to provide him with notification of local epidemics of certain diseases and quarterly figures concerning vaccination.[37] It was also Simon who prevailed upon Parliament to require the GRO to produce the first *Decennial Supplement* of mortality data, covering the period 1851 to 1860.[38] Finally, in the late-1860s Simon persuaded the GRO to enlarge the quarterly returns to include details of the causes and numbers of deaths in subdistricts.[39]

But in order to convert this growing pressure for medical statistics into resources for the Statistical Department, the GRO needed to have the trust and support of the Treasury. That the Office was able to achieve this was not due to William Farr but to the abilities and energy of his superior, Major George Graham. Graham, who was

Registrar General from 1842 to 1879, was born in 1801, the younger son of an important landed family in Cumberland, and the brother of Sir James Graham, the Conservative Home Secretary from 1841 to 1846. He entered the East India Company Service, and retired as a Major in 1831, having been military secretary in Bombay between 1828 and 1830. Graham became private secretary to his brother on the latter's appointment as Home Secretary in the Peel Ministry, and was appointed Registrar General, presumably via his kinsman's influence, on the death of Thomas Lister in 1842.[40] Graham has been overshadowed almost completely by his subordinate, William Farr. Those historians who have noted his existence have tended to regard him as either a weak figure,[41] or as a capable but dull administrator who contented himself with providing Farr with the tools for his statistical work.[42] This is hardly the figure who emerges from an analysis of the extant administrative record, and a good case can be made for the success, and much of the élan, of the GRO in the early Victorian period as being the product of his character and abilities.

When Graham took over the GRO in 1842 he found it in chaos. The lax administration of Thomas Lister had brought the Office to the brink of collapse. The compilation of the registers of births, marriages and deaths was years in arrears, and the office accounts in a disorganised state.[43] Many of the members of staff had been wrongly paid, and some had been swindling the Office.[44] The Audit Office and the Treasury were plainly concerned about the running of the department. Graham's actions were swift and decisive. Offending members of staff were dismissed; task work was introduced to cut backlogs; and the amount of writing reduced by the simple expedient of providing pre-printed pro-forma register entries with gaps for the clerks to fill in.[45] The Treasury expressed itself pleased with Graham's work in turning the Office round, and he gained a reputation for efficiency which stood him in good stead when he asked for staff increases in the 1840s and 1850s.[46] He continued to work ceaselessly to improve the working of the registration system; introducing travelling inspectors to supervise the local registrars; organising the administration of the census; and maintaining discipline in what was often a fractious department.[47] William Farr plainly regarded him highly, commenting at the time of his retirement that

> For more than 37 years I have had the pleasure to serve under Major Graham, and had constant cause to admire and respect the energy, ability, personal attention to details, and capacity for organisation which marked his successful control of civil registration. No one

acquainted with his duties, or with the way in which they were performed by Major Graham, can either describe his post as a sinecure or refuse to recognise the value of the services of the late Registrar General, although of a distinctly different character to my statistical duties.[48]

The gradual expansion of the GRO's statistical manpower enabled Farr to undertake the epidemiological and sanitary research for which the GRO became justly famous.[49]

The years of decline and recovery, 1880 to 1920

As already noted, the two decades after the retirement of Farr and Graham in 1879 were a period when the *Annual Reports of the Registrar General* entered a period of relative decline. As documents they were both shorter and more standardised than those of the earlier period. In a seminal article on the GRO, Simon Szreter has defended the GRO's statistical superintendents in these years, William Ogle and John Tatham, as men of learning, intellectual curiosity and innovation.[50] Rather than a product of deficiencies in scientific personnel, he sees the malaise in the Office of this period as due to three main causes. The GRO's provision of localised mortality statistics had become scientifically outmoded because of the rise of the germ theory, and of social darwinism and eugenics, which down graded the importance of the environmentalism inherent in the Victorian public health movement; increased financial stringency, 'heralded with a Treasury minute of 1886, inaugurating a regime of inflexibility and refusal to countenance expansion in staff costs or improvements in pay'; and the differing personal styles of the successive Registrar Generals and their statistical superintendents.[51] These points need to be considered in turn.

Szreter has recently elaborated his argument with respect to the intellectual cul-de-sac in which the GRO found itself in the late nineteenth century in a major work, *Fertility, Class and Gender in Britain 1860-1940*. Here he portrays the environmentalist credo of the public health movement as under sustained attack from the eugenic theories of men such as Francis Galton and Karl Pearson. Why improve local environmental conditions if this only allowed the unfit to breed sick children?[52] He implies that the rebirth of the GRO's intellectual, and presumably its publishing, endeavours in the early twentieth century reflected the resurgence of environmentalist thinking. This he identifies in turn with the elaboration of the concept of social class differentiation as a mechanism for reproducing cultural and economic deprivation from generation to generation. The GRO is seen as contributing to this revival by elaborating for the 1911 census the socio-economic classification of families, based on the occupation of the male household head, which has been so central to research in the social sciences ever since.[53] In this the GRO was, he argues, feeding directly into the new environmentalism being espoused by Arthur Newsholme, the chief medical officer of health at the Local Government Board from 1908 onwards, in opposition to the eugenicists. Newsholme had a close working relationship with T H C Stevenson, the GRO's superintendent of statistics from 1909 onwards and the author of its model of socio-economic groupings.[54]

This is an extremely imposing explanatory model, supported by a wealth of evidence. It is somewhat difficult, however, to apply it directly to explain the changing form of the *Annual Reports* over time. What were the specific events in the late 1870s which took the wind out the GRO's sails, and what constellation of events in the late-1890s led to the expansion of its output in the new century? Similarly, why exactly should the statistical project of the GRO wind down in these circumstances? After all, and as Szreter stresses, there was a growing demand for data by the increasingly professional and influential body of medical officers of health.[55] Also, the field of aggregate mortality statistics was one in which the GRO could, and did, score vital points for the environmentalist cause. The first mention of eugenic arguments in the *Annual Reports* was as early as that for 1879. The then Registrar General, Brydges Henniker, on noting an apparent recent rise in mortality rates amongst the middle aged and elderly, as opposed to steady improvements amongst younger age cohorts, commented that:

> it has been suggested that it is to sanitation that the increased death-rates of persons after a certain age should be referred. A vast number of children of permanently unsound constitution, are, it is said, now saved from death by sanitary interference. These grow up to adult life, and by their presence diminish the average healthiness of the adult classes, and so add to their death-rates.[56]

Henniker was able to dispose of this argument by noting that sanitation would save the lives of people at all ages, and that one would therefore expect rising mortality in all age cohorts, not just those over 45, if the eugenic model was correct. Also the mortality rates for the elderly now seemed to be improving, which again did not square with eugenic arguments.[57] If eugenics could be so easily dismissed in the early 1880s, why should it lead to the sudden curtailment of the GRO's publishing activities at this date?

Similarly, why should the rise of biological germ theories of disease causation undermine aggregate statistical production? After all, William Farr himself came to believe in germs as biological entities which caused disease.[58] Laboratory based medicine does not appear to have undermined statistical epidemiology in the period after 1900. This is clearly seen in the research infrastructure set up by the Medical Research Committee, the precursor of the Medical Research Council, in 1914. This was made up of three departments of experimental research (bacteriology, biochemistry and pharmacology, and applied physiology), plus a Statistical Department under John Brownlee.[59] A perusal of the latter's publications at this date reveals him to be undertaking statistical epidemiological research bearing a striking resemblance to that traditionally undertaken by the GRO.[60] Aggregate data was still required, although it might need to be interpreted in a different manner.

Szreter's arguments with respect to the financial and staffing problems of the GRO are equally difficult to interpret. It should be noted at the outset that the secondary sources he draws on here relate to the Local Government Board, rather than to the GRO directly.[61] As can be seen from Figure 3, the GRO did indeed have staffing problems in the late Victorian period. The underlying causes of this are twofold.[62] First, in the 1870s and 1880s the Treasury insisted that there should be no more recruitment into the Office until existing members of staff had been promoted over time to new Civil Service grades then being introduced.[63] Secondly, in 1889 the Treasury insisted on increasing the working day in the GRO, in line with the rest of the Civil Service, from six to seven hours, with consequential reductions in the numbers of staff. This was particularly serious in an office where so much work was done on overtime.[64] With the population expanding throughout this period, the GRO's staffing problems must have caused increasing difficulties with respect to the processing of certificates of registration.

However, as can be seen from Table 3.1 (p. 71), the Statistical Department does not appear to have suffered in the same manner as the rest of the Office from stagnant or falling staffing levels. The main staffing problems appear to have been in the Records Department which dealt with the compilation of the registers used by the public to obtain proof of birth, marriage or death. In addition, the period from 1870 onwards was marked by the introduction into the GRO of new computational technology, in the form of arithmometers, comptometers, and slide rules, expressly with the aim of boosting the productivity of the statistical clerks.[65] The argument that financial stringency underlay the publishing malaise of the GRO in the last two decades of the Victorian period is thus somewhat difficult to prove.

It might be appropriate at this point, therefore, to turn to the third factor which Szreter adduces to explain the relative decline of the GRO – the replacement of the Office's senior personnel in 1880. He sees this as a trigger for the expression of the underlying forces of change discussed above. But if the underlying forces he cites are problematic, or do not appear to fit the chronology of decline, does the trigger not become a more substantive factor in its own right? Perhaps rather than equating the history of the GRO with the superintendents of statistics, Ogle and Tatham, one should consider the role of the Registrar General in the period 1880 to 1900, Brydges Henniker. If there was a malaise within the GRO in this period, a good case can be made for seeing it as stemming from its administrative head.

Brydges Henniker was born in 1835, son of Sir Augustus Brydges Henniker and cousin of Lord Henniker, and succeeded to his father's baronetcy in 1849. He served in the 68th Foot and the Horse Guards and was also captain in the West Essex Yeomanry. He was appointed head of the GRO in 1880 by George Sclater-Booth, President of the Local Government Board, under whom he was serving as private secretary.[66] Compared to Graham, Henniker seems to have been a less forceful and competent administrator. His correspondence with the Treasury is much sparser, and far less confrontational. There appears to have been only one occasion in 20 years on which Henniker actually asked the Treasury for more staff, and much of the increasing workload of the office came to be performed on overtime.[67] By the end of Henniker's period of office, the Treasury itself had become alarmed at the hours that men in the GRO were working.[68] Nor was he as ready as Graham to fight for better remuneration for his staff, a situation which led in 1885 to his clerks asking independently for a commission of inquiry into pay.[69] At this point the Treasury asked that in future Henniker should pass all important staffing matters through the Local Government Board but the latter declined to take on the responsibility.[70] Henniker was also far more likely to seek guidance from his parent department as to the running of the registration system, a habit which on occasion caused exasperation amongst the Board's officers.[71] It is possible, therefore, that the loss of nerve within the GRO in the 1880s and 1890s reflected failings at the top of the organisation.

Certainly, Henniker's removal from the scene led to a sudden burst of re-organisation within the Office. In 1899 whilst he was still Registrar General but absent through illness, the assistant Registrar General, Noel Humphreys, was asking for, and obtaining, additional staff.[72] In the early years of the next decade two quite short-lived departmental heads, Sir Reginald MacLeod (1900–02) and Sir William Cospatrick Dunbar (1902–09), successfully expanded the staff of the Office, especially via the introduction of women clerks and typists.[73] This included the establishment of the first permanent census unit within the GRO, comprising three clerks, in 1904.[74]

Changes in the form of the *Annual Report* were closely linked to Henniker's period of office. In his first *Report* he printed Farr's final, and very brief Letter.[75] But in his second annual publication the Letter disappeared, or rather was absorbed into the Registrar General's text.[76] The size of Henniker's own contribution began to shrink rapidly, declining from 43 pages in 1880 to 18 pages in 1884.[77] During his brief spell as Registrar General, MacLeod continued the form of Henniker's *Annual Reports*. However, his successor, Dunbar, immediately reinstated the superintendent of statistic's Letter in 1903.[78] The reason Dunbar gave for doing so was not linked to the needs of the Local Government Board, or of medical officers of health, rather he claimed:

> I have adopted this course as it occurs to me that the medical practitioners of this country, on whose generous co-operation the accurate compilation of vital statistics so largely depends, will, in this way, more readily appreciate the fact that the particulars they contribute concerning the causes of death are analysed, and the results authenticated, by a member of their own profession.[79]

This change was, of course, introduced some years before either Newsholme or Stevenson took up their respective posts in the Local Government Board and the GRO.

The tentative conclusion to be drawn from this analysis, is that it is somewhat difficult to argue conclusively for the chronology of changes in the form of the *Annual Reports* in the late nineteenth and early twentieth centuries in terms of intellectual history or of finance. A much simpler explanation, that of the key role of the respective Registrar Generals, seems just as likely. Perhaps there has been a tendency to look for profound and momentous scientific changes to explain something rather trivial and mundane.

Anonymity, 1920

Szreter's discussion of the sudden anonymisation of the *Annual Reports* in 1920, and their replacement by the *Registrar General's*

Statistical Review thereafter, also reflects the priority he gives to broad predisposing factors rather than to the internal politics of Whitehall. He stresses the rise of a professional cadre of medical officers of health as undermining the GRO's commitment to wider public education, so that

> By the end of the Great War the GRO had ceased altogether to reflect in the style of its publications the 'democratic' and libertarian values that were the central core of its operational philosophy in the founding era of Farr and Graham. The adoption of an entirely anonymous format in its publications from 1920 succinctly conveys this more purely bureaucratic and authoritarian ethos.[80]

But this development was not, it will be argued here, a development internal to the GRO, or due to changes in local government. Rather, 1920 marks the sudden and abrupt end of the relative constitutional independence of the GRO, with the subordination of the Office to the Ministry of Health. The new ethos of the GRO reflected how the Ministry saw its proper functions rather than a gradual internal metamorphosis within the GRO.

At its inception in the 1830s the GRO was only notionally responsible to the Home Office. Under the 1836 Registration Act the Registrar General was directly appointed by the Crown, and negotiated directly with the Treasury over the staffing of his department. As already discussed, after the GRO passed under the ministerial responsibility of the President of the Local Government Board in 1871, the latter does not appear to have wished to alter the essential nature of these arrangements. The Ministry of Health, under which the GRO passed in 1919, had a very different concept of the proper relationship between itself and its subordinate agencies. Following the recommendations of the Haldane Committee, the Minister of Health, Addison, had a vision of a department within which the research was integrated with policy making.[81] The aim of the Ministry in its dealings with the GRO became the subordination of the latter to policy making.

In order to achieve this, the Ministry installed Sylvanus Vivian as deputy Registrar General. Vivian had worked at the National Health Insurance Commission under Sir Robert Morant, who later became the first permanent secretary of the Ministry of Health.[82] Vivian became the real power within the GRO, forming the conduit for all negotiations with the Ministry and Treasury over the organisation of the Office.[83] His first task after being appointed in November 1919 was 'to examine the organisation of the department and to report thereon to the Director of Establishment [of the Ministry].' The

Registrar General, Sir Bernard Mallet, was merely to be 'informed of all proposals and developments'.[84] Mallet was so incensed by being sidelined in this manner that he eventually resigned in 1920, to be succeeded by Vivian.

Vivian's views on the proper role of the GRO's Statistical Department reflected the Ministry's stance. In a memorandum of 1920 entitled, 'Registrar General's Department. Memorandum on re-organisation of duties', he declared:

> The Registrar General's Department must not be the Department responsible for initiating or originating research upon its statistics; for if it did so on its own initiative it might be duplicating, or cutting across the work of other departments properly charged with such duties. In order that it may be suitably guided and advised by its clients, the other departments of the Ministry and other government departments and public organisations which utilise its products, there should be a standing statistical council within the Ministry, comprising representatives of all the clients referred to. The duty of this Council would be to focus the requirements of all departments and bodies, to reconcile them if incompatible, and to present them to the Registrar General's department by way of advice as to the particular items of information which (subject to administrative considerations) ought to be collected, and as to the shape and manner generally in which the statistics could most usefully be presented.[85]

It was most probably the imposition of this perception of the ancillary role of the GRO, rather than any internal cultural changes, which led to the alterations in the form of the *Annual Report* in 1920.

Conclusions

The arguments rehearsed here are perhaps somewhat unfair to those, such as Simon Szreter, who have attempted to explain changes in the GRO's published output in terms of deep-seated scientific and cultural developments. It is very seldom that one finds documentary evidence which could prove such links conclusively. This applies equally to the present article – there is, for example, no textual evidence that the views of the Ministry of Health on the proper role of the GRO led directly to the imposition of anonymity in the GRO's publications in 1920. There is no sources which can act as a 'smoking gun'. All that can be argued is that the story told here appears to fit the observed phenomena more consistently, and somewhat more economically.

Also, many of the aspects of Szreter's arguments can indeed be sharpened by the introduction of agency outlined in the present work. Staffing problems may possibly have constrained the GRO in the late Victorian period but this can be seen in terms of the relationship between the Registrar General and the Treasury. The imposition of anonymity in the GRO's publications in 1920 may have reflected bureaucratisation, but this reflected struggles within Whitehall, rather than a disembodied cultural transformation. Institutional and political factors need to be combined with intellectual history to give a fuller picture of the changing nature of the work of the GRO.

Figure 3.1

Delays in publishing the Annual Report of the Registrar General

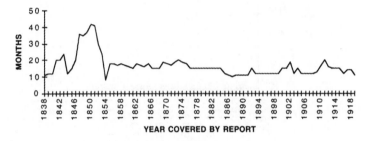

Figure 3.2

Pages of text in the Annual Report of the Registrar General

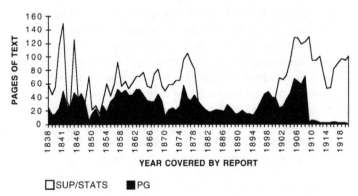

□SUP/STATS ■PG

Note: the area shaded black represents the pages of the Registrar General's own report; the area between this and the top line represents the pages of the superintendent of statistic's letter. The whole area below the top line represents the cumulative pages in the *Annual Report* of that year.

69

Figure 3.3
Staffing of the GRO

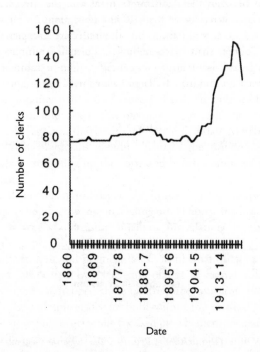

Date

Note: This graph includes all clerical and senior staff of the GRO, plus transcribers, indexers, abstractors, copyists and sorters. It excludes industrial grades and typists. Prior to the estimates for 1860, transcribers, indexers, abstractors, copyists and sorters were not included. From 1889-90 copyists were not included in the estimates – number based therefore on the amount of money spent on copyists in 1888-89 (£2,740) divided by number of copyists (21) to give an average cost of a copyist (£130). This is then used to calculate the number of notional copyists in later years by dividing the amount spent on copyists by this figure.

Sources: Civil Service Estimates

Table 3.1
GRO Staffing 1840–1921

Department

Date	Correspondence[1]	Accounts	Records	Statistics	Total[2]
1840	10	6	29	4	50
1842 (April)	10	5	50	8	74
1842 (July)	—	—	—	—	87
1843	—	—	—	—	60
1855	—	—	—	—	70
1864	—	—	—	—	78
1866	4	4	50	16	78
1874	—	—	—	—	78
1895	—	11	45	19	78
1905	—	—	—	27	84
1912/1913	—	—	—	—	103
1921	—	9	114	48	172[3]

Notes:

1   The Correspondence Branch was amalgamated with Accounts after 1866.

2   Includes Registrar General, heads of departments and inspectors of registration but excludes industrial grades.

3   Excludes 38 typists.

Sources: 1840, Imperial Calendar; 1842(Apr), RG 29/1, pp 119-141; 1842(July), RG 29/1, pp 202; 1843, RG 29/1, pp 202; 1855, RG 29/5, p 385 (pp 3-4); 1864, RG 29/6, pp 9-10; 1866, RG 29/2, pp 54-5; 1874, RG 29/2, p 184; 1895, T1/8954A/13154; 1905, RG 20/74; 1912-13, T 165/40; 1921, RG 20/81

Notes

1. The research on which this paper is based was undertaken whilst the author was a Wellcome research fellow at the Wellcome Unit for the History of Medicine, Oxford.

2. The main works on the history of the GRO in the period under consideration here are: John M Eyler, *Victorian Social Medicine. The Ideas and Methods of William Farr* (Baltimore and London: Johns Hopkins University Press, 1979); Muriel Nissel, *People Count. A History of the General Register Office* (London: HMSO, 1987); Simon Szreter, 'The GRO and the public health movement in Britain 1837-1914,' *Social History of Medicine* 4 (1991), 435–63; Simon Szreter, *Fertility, Class and Gender in Britain 1860-1940* (Cambridge: Cambridge University Press, 1996).

3. For the history of the GRO's involvement with the census see, Edward Higgs, *Making Sense of the Census. The Manuscript Returns for England and Wales, 1801-1901* (London: HMSO, 1989), 2-16.

4. See, for example, Ian Hacking, *The Emergence of Probability* (Cambridge: Cambridge University Press, 1975); Theodore M. Porter, *The Rise of Statistical Thinking 1820-1900* (Princeton: Princeton University Press, 1986); Stephen M. Stigler, *The History of Statistics: The Measurement of Uncertainty Before 1900* (Cambridge, Mass.: Belknap Press of Harvard University Press, 1986); Lorraine Daston, *Classical Probability in the Enlightenment* (Princeton: Princeton University Press, 1988); Ian Hacking, *The Taming of Chance* (Cambridge: Cambridge University Press, 1990); J. Rosser Matthews, *Quantification and the Quest for Medical Certainty* (Princeton: Princeton University Press, 1995).

5. This is an excerpt from William Farr's presidential address to the Statistical Society of London, 1872, quoted in: Eyler, *op. cit.* (note 2), 28.

6. For Farr's approach to statistics see Eyler, *op. cit.* (note 2), *passim.*

7. For this development, see Donald A. MacKenzie, *Statistics in Britain, 1865-1930. The Social Construction of Scientific Knowledge* (Edinburgh: Edinburgh University Press, 1981), as well as the texts cited in note 4 above.

8. For Quetelet's concept of the 'homme moyen' see, Daston, *op. cit.* (note 4), 381–5.

9. Eyler, *op. cit.* (note 2), 28.

10. Notable exceptions have been: Simon Szreter, 'The GRO and the public health movement in Britain 1837-1914', *Social History of Medicine* 4 (1991), 435–464: 438–9, 454–5; Anne Hardy, 'Death is

the end of all disease: using the GRO cause of death statistics for 1837-1920', *Social History of Medicine* 7 (1994), 472–92: 473–4.

11. It included more questions than the 1841 enumeration and covered groups excluded from the earlier enumeration, such as those aboard ships and those sleeping rough. The population census was also associated with a census of facilities for religious worship and for education.

12. Parliamentary Papers (hereafter PP) 1850 XX-1 [1255.]

13. *11th Annual Report of the Registrar General* (hereafter *ARRG*) *for 1848* (London, 1852), i.

14. Hardy alludes to this problem: Hardy, *op. cit.* (note 10), 474, n.7. In the present work all references are made to the complete versions of the *Annual Reports* rather than to Parliamentary Papers.

15. This graph relates solely to the textual commentary on the published tables but this can be taken as indicative of the GRO's commitment to a public propaganda role.

16. This appears to have been especially the case in the 1840s when the *7th, 9th, 10th Annual Reports* do not contain a Letter from the superintendent of statistics: *7th ARRG for 1843 and 1844* (London, 1846); *9th ARRG for 1846* (London, 1849); *10th ARRG for 1847* (London, 1852). These problems are noted by Hardy, *op. cit.* (note 10), 474. She claims, however, that there was no cause of death information published between 1848 and 1855, which is incorrect: see *12th ARRG for 1849* (London, 1853), 252–69; *13th ARRG for 1850* (London, 1854), 150–67; *14th ARRG for 1851* (London, 1855), 120–37; *15th ARRG for 1852* (London, 1855), 122–41; *16th ARRG for 1853* (London, 1856), 124–39: *17th ARRG for 1854* (London, 1856), 120–39. There are also summaries of the quarterly returns in all these reports.

17. Szreter, *op. cit.* (note 10), 454.

18. *64th ARRG for 1901* (London, 1903).

19. *72nd ARRG for 1909* (London, 1911).

20. *83rd ARRG for 1920* (London, 1922).

21. *Registrar General's Statistical Review for 1921* (London, 1923).

22. The *Annual Reports* in these years were not only shorter than those of the 1860s and 1870s but had a formulaic air. Indeed, some of the *Reports* in this period merely repeated the wording of previous *Reports* with different dates and numbers inserted.

23. The *Annual Reports* did not, of course, exhaust the GRO's published output. By 1840 the GRO was collecting cause of death data from the Metropolitan registrars on a weekly basis, and publishing an abstract of the information. From the mid-1860s similar material

was published for ten large provincial towns, and the numbers so covered increased during the course of Victoria's reign. As already noted, from 1842 the Office published quarterly reports on general mortality rates in 114 of the most populous districts of the country. A new quarterly series covering all registration districts began in 1849, and in 1870 these were upgraded to give cause of death. In 1864, Farr published a supplement to the *Annual Report* in which he summarised the mortality experience of England and Wales in the two decades 1841-50 and 1851-60. The *Decennial Supplement* then became a standard periodic feature of the GRO's output.

24. Edward Higgs, 'A cuckoo in the nest? The origins of civil registration and state medical statistics in England and Wales', *Continuity and Change* 11 (1996), 115–34; 115–26.

25. 6 & 7 Will IV c 86 s vi.

26. *1st ARRG for the year ending 30 June 1838* (London: 1839), Appendix P, 65–125.

27. Higgs, *op. cit.* (note 24), 126–30.

28. *Ibid.*, 123.

29. 11 & 12 Vict., c.63.

30. Szreter, *op. cit.* (note 10), 439–40. It should be noted, however, that as early as 1844, Edwin Chadwick was using data obtained from the GRO to show the differences in the numbers of births and deaths in London which would have resulted if the Metropolis had the same mortality regime as Hereford: Edwin Chadwick, 'On the best modes of representing accurately, by statistical returns, the duration of life, and the pressure and progress of the causes of mortality amongst different classes of the community, and amongst the population of different districts and countries', *Journal of the Statistical Society of London*, 7 (1844), 16–17.

31. Public Record Office (hereafter PRO): General Register Office Letter Books (RG 29): RG 29/2, 128.

32. PRO: RG 29/1, 246. The Treasury agreed to this request in March of that year: PRO: RG 29/5, 267–8.

33. PRO: General Board of Health: Correspondence (MH 13): MH 13/260.

34. PRO: MH 13/260, letters of 9 May and 22 June 1855.

35. Royston Lambert, *Sir John Simon and English social administration 1816-1904* (London: MacGibbon & Kee, 1963), 262–3.

36. *Papers Relating to the Sanitary State of the People of England* (London, 1858; reprinted Farnborough: Gregg, 1973).

37. *1st Report of the Medical Officer of the Privy Council*, PP 1859, XII [257.], 279–81.

38. *4th Report of the Medical Officer of the Privy Council,* PP 1862, XXII [465.], 500-1; a copy of the Parliamentary order, dated 24 July 1863, can be found in PRO: Treasury Board Papers (T 1): T 1/6452A/17223.

39. *1st Report of the Royal Sanitary Commission,* PP 1868-9, XXXII [301.], QQ 1908-10; *2nd Report of the Royal Sanitary Commission,* PP 1871 XXXV [c.231], Q 9695; *11th Report of the Medical Officer of the Privy Council,* PP 1868-9, XXXII [1.], 23.

40. Nissel, *op. cit.* (note 2), 147.

41. Lambert, *op. cit.* (note 35), 419.

42. On the basis of two letters from Graham to Farr which survive in the Farr papers, Eyler concludes that 'Graham was slow to make changes, reluctant to put pressure on the government, and interested in guaranteeing the accomplishment of routine tasks': Eyler, *op. cit.* (note 2), 49.

43. PRO: RG 29/1, 177; RG 29/5, 186.

44. PRO: RG 29/1, 210-2, 229–30.

45. PRO: RG 29/1, 183–4.

46. PRO: RG 29/5, 219.

47. PRO: RG 29/1, 209; RG 29/5, 229.

48. *The Times,* 20 January 1880, 8.

49. For the range of Farr's activities see, Eyler, *op. cit.* (note 2), *passim.*

50. Szreter, *op. cit.* (note 10), 457–60.

51. *Ibid.,* 455–7.

52. Simon Szreter, *Fertility, Class and Gender in Britain 1860-1940* (Cambridge: Cambridge University Press, 1996), 93–107.

53. Szreter, *op. cit.* (note 10), 458–62; Szreter, *op. cit.* (note 52), 182–237.

54. *Ibid.,* 238–53.

55. *Ibid.,* 197–203.

56. *42nd ARRG for 1879* (London, 1881), xxiii.

57. *Ibid.,* xxiii–xxiv.

58. Eyler, *op. cit.* (note 2), 106–7.

59. A. Landsborough Thomson, *Half a Century of Medical Research. Volume 1: Origins and Policy of the Medical Research Council (UK)* (London: HMSO, 1973), 110.

60. PRO: Annual Reports of the MRC (FD 2): FD 2/1 First Annual Report of the Medical Research Committee, 1914–1915, p. 23.

61. Szreter, *op. cit.* (note 10), 455, n.78. He is referring to the work of Roy MacLeod: 'The frustration of state medicine', *Medical History* 11 (1967), 15–40; Roy MacLeod, *Treasury Control and Social Administration* (London: Bell, 1968).

62. The Treasury memorandum of 1886 which Szreter cites appears to have been a fairly standard circular to departments which was not itself a key factor in the GRO's staffing difficulties.

63. PRO: RG 29/2, 107–9, 375–6 (insert).

64. PRO: RG 29/7, pp 21–23, 37; PRO: RG 29/3, 64.

65. Edward Higgs, 'The statistical Big Bang of 1911: ideology, technological innovation and the production of medical statistics', *Social History of Medicine* 9 (1996), 409–26.

66. *The Times*, 8 January 1880, 11.

67. PRO: RG 29/2, 335–6.

68. PRO: RG 29/7, 134.

69. PRO: RG 29/2, 356–78.

70. PRO: RG 29/6, 282, 284.

71. PRO: Local Government Board Correspondence (MH 19): MH 19/194, correspondence dated 16 January 1882, 14 December 1886; PRO: MH 19/195, correspondence dated, 11 May 1891.

72. PRO: RG 29/3, 236; PRO: RG 29/7, 143.

73. PRO: RG 29/3, 266, 273, 280, 348; PRO: RG 29/7, 163, 167, 171–4, 182, 201–2.

74. PRO: RG 29/3, 310; PRO: RG 29/7, 184.

75. *41st ARRG for 1878* (London, 1880).

76. *42nd ARRG for 1879* (London, 1881).

77. *41st ARRG for 1878* (London, 1880), v–xlviii; *45th ARRG for 1882* (London, 1884), v–xxiii.

78. *64th ARRG for 1901* (London, 1903), xxx–lxxiv.

79. *Ibid.*, xxi.

80. Szreter, *op. cit.* (note 10), 453.

81. Steven Stacey, 'The Ministry of Health 1919-1929: ideas and practice in a government department', D. Phil Thesis, Oxford, 1984, 12, 49–50.

82. *Ibid.*, 43.

83. PRO: Ministry of Health and Predecessors and Successors: Establishment and Organisation Files (MH 78): MH 78/114 General Register Office co-ordination of work with Ministry of Health and appointment of Registrar General: memo of 7/11/1919; Note of Dr Addison's. Discussion of Registrar General's Department.

84. PRO: MH 78/114, memo of 7/11/1919.

85. PRO: MH 78/114, Registrar General's Department. Memorandum on re-organisation of duties. The internal Ministry committee never materialised but the Statistical Committee of the Medical Research Council came to fulfil the same function in the course of the 1920s.

4

Metrological Awakenings:
Rationalising the Body Electric in
Nineteenth-Century Medicine

John Senior

Quantitative reasoning in electrotherapy was a controversial issue as emerging new electrical technologies and medical science converged in the embryonic discipline of neurology in Britain between 1860-1920. Before the Society of Telegraph Engineers in 1882, William Stone (1830-91), a medical electrician at St. Thomas's Hospital, warned that his specialty had suffered from too exclusive handling by medical men and physiologists:

> Medicine and its kindred arts lend themselves ill to measurement; the tone of mind required for the practice is rather judicial than computative; it is oftener concerned with weighing evidence, and balancing alternatives than with solving equations.[1]

Four years later his colleague, Armand De Watteville (1846-1925), head of St. Mary's Electrical Department, wrote equally disparagingly about contemporary developments in electrotherapy in his review of C. W. Müller's *Introduction to Elektrotherapie*:

> The author takes the same standpoint which we ourselves have always assumed, *viz.* that the fundamental question in electrical treatment is one of physics, and not of physiology. It is with much satisfaction that we see the question of current measurement occupy a more and more prominent position in the various papers and books published on this subject and the unit we first proposed 'milliweber or milliampere' adopted by all good observers.[2]

For both these medical electricians, neither greater clinical acumen nor deeper physiological understanding would bring them any closer to a rational therapy based on standardised dosages of electricity and conciliation of theory and practice. The role of quantification in medical reasoning had been subordinated to the exercise of clinical judgment, and until the exact methods of physics could be deployed, practice would remain forever empirical. I will argue, however, that such quantitative strategies based on instrumentation (mainly the galvanometer) to standardise electrotherapy led not to greater therapeutic certainty but its impediment. By paying attention to such metrological considerations as current strength and dosage, medical electricians focussed attention on the electrical resistivity of the body. The application of Ohm's Law to the body, however, yielded conflicting measurements and limitations of engineering the body to conform to electromedical standards.

The image of the doctor as engineer was controversial in Victorian England. Electricity had diverse and incompatible associations with all aspects of society – popular remedies, such as the electric belt, industry and communications. Moreover, technology and specialism often provoked hostile attitudes among conservative members of the medical profession, for it conflicted with the gentlemanly ideal of a liberally educated doctor groomed in the clinic rather than in the laboratory.[3] Skeptical medical practitioners often disclaimed electrotherapy on the grounds of therapeutic error, of patient suggestion and natural remission of disease.

Fittingly, perhaps, from the early Victorian period onward, textbook writers on natural philosophy such as Golding Bird and Charles Brooke viewed electrotherapeutics as the exemplar of the utility of science in medicine.[4] Electromedical advocates successfully fostered treatments comprised principally of Galvanism, the application of a continuous current from a battery, and Faradism, the application of an interrupted current from the induction coil or dynamo, initially in specialised hospitals for nervous disease and paralysis such as the National Hospital, Queen Square, founded in 1860, and later in electrotherapeutic departments in general hospitals.

The plausibility of electrotherapy was founded within the growing reductionist tendencies of physiology in the first half of the nineteenth century. In 1846 William Grove, in his *Correlation of Physical Forces,* showed that the body was the site of the conservation of energy principle in which all physical and biological forces were viewed as a manifestation of a universal energy that could not be created nor destroyed and was, thus, subject to measurement.[5] In the latter half of the nineteenth century, the American, George M. Beard coined the term 'neurasthenia' and joined commentators in viewing fatigue as an elaboration of the second law of thermodynamics (*i.e.,* entropy of the universe tends towards a maximum). The same dynamical forces that governed the productivity and efficiency of machinery were seen at play in the body in motion.[6] Electrical circuits prevailed in the body as well as in technological devices. Neurasthenia revealed itself in the form of the body's battery run down.

Plausibility also came in the guise of the electrical telegraph. Just as in the nineteenth century the telegraph cable linked Lord Kelvin's vision of industry and empire, so the body too was analogically colonialised by the telegraph cable of the electrical engineer. Paralysed patients and epileptics were viewed by medical electricians in terms of the body's defective telegraph system. Electricity could be applied to detect and repair the body's communication system arranged according to the reticular nervous system.

The body was construed as a system of connections in which the technological reification of the concept of circulation (of electricity or of nervous force) allowed the distinction between the organic and the mechanical to be blurred.[7] Yet concern about electricity's problematic relationship with the nervous force throughout the century belied medical electricians' strict adherence to reductionism. Shot through electrotherapy was an 'electrovitalism' that retarded the development of electrotherapy as the paradigmatic example of the 'new physiological therapeutics' in which qualitative descriptions of the natural were replaced by abstract numerical and visual elaboration of the normal.[8] Not that electricity's grand polar properties of attraction and repulsion, stimulation and sedation, plus its dual function as a diagnostic and therapeutic agent, were construed as an all-important cosmological principle that stood in antithesis to orthodox medicine. As Cooter points out, under the banner of organicism, such polar doctrines connoting wholeness, harmony and unity subsumed mechanism instead of construing reality analogically in terms of contradictory opposites in dialectical relation.[9] The dichotomy between alternative and orthodox practices, in fact, became less and less apparent as 'alternative' medical electricians like Harry Lobb, founder of the Galvanic Hospital, were orthodox trained and defended their theories and practices on the terrain of a positivist science.[10] The electrophysiologist C. B. Radcliffe at the National Hospital, Queen Square, found support in W. R. Grove's *On the Correlation of Physical Forces* for his anti-reductionist beliefs in the unity of nature by deploying the allegory of the Proteus myth.[11] A correlation of physical and vital forces allowed practitioners to emphasise practice over theory.[12] Such methodological imprecision enabled practitioners to refer to measuring the nervous force without any reference to electricity until well into the twentieth century.[13]

Rather than the spectre of materialism, however, the fear haunting electromedicine at the end of the century was that of the 'dementalising of the physician' – a term used by the American neurologist Silas Weir Mitchell to describe a kind of de-skilling caused by technology.[14] The reluctance to replace qualitative descriptions of the natural with the abstract and numerical of instrumentation was evident, for example, in the first so-called clinical trial of electricity conducted by members of the Royal Medical and Chirurgical Society (RMCS) in 1865–68.[15] The minutes record attention being paid to standardising equipment but not to dosage. Galvanometry was eschewed in favour of the phenomenological characteristics of electrical output such as 'the different results to be obtained from the induction current of the ordinary kind and the continuous current rapidly interrupted ... the different effects obtained from a few large plates and a large number of small plates [electrostatic generator].'[16] In describing the superior qualities of the Becker-Muirhead battery for the treatment of neurosis, a member of the RMCS team, Julius Althaus (1833-1900), later wrote that 'one 1/12 increment of intensity produced sensations that were hardly perceptible on the tongue and face and all intermediate degrees up to a point which would not be relished by the most hardened garrotta.'[17]

Althaus, a founder of the Maida Vale Hospital for Epilepsy and Paralysis (1866), had been commissioned by the editors of the *British Medical Journal* to review the current state of electromedical apparatus. In doing so he precipitated debate about technology and the 'dementalising of the physician.' It pitched proponents of metrology against those who questioned the substitution of clinical experience with the so-called precision of instrumentation. On the one side stood the 'progressives,' John Dixon Mann (1840-1912), a notable Manchester physician, and Armand de Watteville of St. Mary's University College Hospital, and on the other side, Herbert Tibbits (fl. 1860), Medical Superintendent of the National Hospital, Queen Square. The opening shots were fired by Mann in a note to the *Lancet* in 1877. He had observed that greater precision of late had been given to the administration of electricity through a deeper scientific understanding of electrical apparatus.[18] Agreeing with Althaus's observations in the *British Medical Journal* that the Becker-Muirhead battery provided the most constant current for electrotherapy, Mann went on to assert that an efficient battery should comprise of about 30 to 50 cells. The battery should be fitted with a suitable selector so as to avoid a break during the change in the number of cells in the circuit. Otherwise the patient would experience a disagreeable shock. Most important, however, was that a galvanometer should be fitted to the apparatus, not the type supplied with the battery as these were 'merely a galvanoscope,' but a tangent galvanometer and a resistance coil of 150 to 200 ohms.[19] By determining the electromotive force that would be proportional to the tangent of the angle of deflection of the galvanometer, and taking into consideration that the resistance varied not only between individuals but also in the same individual according to the state of the sweat glands, a greater degree of objectivity in electrotherapy could be achieved than the 'tablespoons' of ordinary medical practice.

Such metrological pronouncements on electrotherapy did not go unnoticed by the aspiring medical electrician, Armand De Watteville. In rather dismissive tones, he responded to Mann's letter, saying that he had found Gaiffe's galvanoscope quite suitable for medical practice. Comprising of a moderate number of turns of fine copper wire and graduated from simultaneous reduced readings on a tangent galvanometer in one ten thousandths of a unit, ranging from one to one hundred and fifty, such an instrument, De Watteville exclaimed, could reveal 'a current of 60, 100, or 150 for five or ten minutes [that] conveys the same exact knowledge as so many grains so many times a day.'[20] The most important practical step that needed to be undertaken, De Watteville claimed, was the adoption of a system of electrical units. Now a medical electrician may use the volt, ohm or farad without any fear of being plunged into abstruse physical speculation, De Watteville reassured his reader. The British Association had promulgated a practical system of units. Just as in using the metric system one did not have to trouble oneself about measurements of the earth's circumference upon which it was based, similarly the volt, ohm or farad could be adopted by the practical electrician: 'the ohm is a coil of wire, the standard of resistance. The volt can be spoken of as we would of horsepower. A properly constructed galvanometer will show the current strength as a watch does the time.'[21]

In the same issue of the *Lancet*, a querulous response to Mann's article appeared from Herbert Tibbits. Tibbits objected to relying on galvanometry to give an accurate measure of electricity.[22] Only clinical experience was the true guide to electrotherapy, and clinical experience dictated that 'no two cases of disease require precisely the same dose of electricity. For people differ greatly in their tolerance of electricity, and the exact strength of current which suffices to produce the desired effect should alone be used, and not exceeded.'[23] The electrician had to rely on the testimony of his own senses, rather than on the galvanometer, when either increasing or decreasing the power of the current. Tibbits implored the reader to take the feelings of the patient into consideration, implying that unnecessary pain was concomitant with ordinary electrotherapeutic practice, where the electrician 'has shifted the responsibility to his galvanometer.'[24]

Mann totally disagreed with Tibbits. Reliance on galvanometry enabled estimates of electricity to be made with unfailing exactitude that would not exceed the amount sufficient to provide the required result. Just as in the administration of anaesthesia, Mann argued, 'it is customary to measure the doses although the inhalation is continued until the desired result is obtained. In nervous affections no visible action is produced by electricity. What then is to guide us in giving the amount of current?'[25] Turning Tibbits' argument on its head, Mann argued that though testing the current on the operator first was occasionally useful, the idea of the operator as a self-referential standard was as unreliable as the variations of conductivity of the operator's own skin 'modifying his perception of the current.'[26] Galvanometry would not inexorably lead to pain and loss of control in the clinical situation, but rather greater control in order that the operator may modify it, 'just as the physician increases or diminishes the use of a drug in accordance with the exigencies of each individual case.'[27] Reliance on galvanometry was no more an abnegation of clinical responsibility than 'a carpenter who, distrusting the estimating power of his own eye, resorts to his two foot rule,' Mann concluded.[28]

At the heart of Tibbits' opposition was resistance to an over-reliance on technology at the expense of clinical experience. He believed that 'there is too much tendency already to an almost mechanical use of electricity in medicine, and my belief that the employment of a so-called infallible guide to dosage would make men even more careless than they are at present.'[29] Galvanometry was deceptive. Though it could measure accurately battery strength, inclusion of the human body always made it unreliable. To underline this apparently moral failing of technology, Tibbits recorded the use of an Elliott's tangent galvanometer one morning and listed the results in his reply to Mann. First, Tibbits showed that merely by the mode of application, whether by means of sponges well moistened in water or sponges with salt water, the galvanometric readings would be affected. Then Tibbits tested a case of facial paralysis with currents from four batteries. The number of cells ranged from 15 to 20, to 10 to 18, respectively. With moistened conductors the positive pole was applied to the facial nerve and the negative applied in succession to the paralysed muscles. With the current strength just sufficient to produce muscular contraction, Tibbits declared that when the current was supplied to his own face the sensation produced by the four currents was about the same. Similarly, with his blindfolded patient, she could not distinguish between them. However, the degrees of deflection of the galvanometer needle read 20°, 42°, 30° and 25°.[30]

Tibbits' letter evoked surprise from Dr Mann. Mann was surprised that Tibbits needed to be told that 'when a galvanometer is included in a circuit closed by the human body, the needle will indicate the strength of current passing through the body precisely as though the circuit was closed by a resistance coil or a length of telegraph wire.'[31] Though Tibbits was correct in drawing attention to the condition of the electrodes on the patient's skin, he was mistaken in thinking that a galvanometer could not gauge the amount of current. 'The strength of the current is equal in all parts of the circuit and is governed by the resistance of the circuit', Mann argued. 'Therefore, if the human body formed part of the circuit, the galvanometer would indicate step by step the quantity of electricity passing through the body in accordance with Ohm's law.[32] With respect to Tibbits' experiments using different batteries, Mann had found, on the contrary, after a long series of investigations, readings that were very constant. Tibbits needed to repeat his experiments, 'not once or twice but many times,' Mann advised.

Mann's and De Watteville's metrological exhortations contrasted sharply with those who appealed to the authority of the body as the ultimate arbiter of dosage. With self-referential assurance, Tibbits stressed to his reader: the importance of always testing electricity upon yourselves before applying it to a patient

> Use as many galvanometers, or so-called 'instruments of precision' as you like, but use in addition the back of your left hand as a convenient approximate test for the voltaic, and your thumb muscles for the faradic current, except when about to apply electricity to your patient's head or face and make it then an invariable rule to first apply to your own face the same strength of current you are about to administer to your patient.[33]

Apportioning greater value to the clinical gaze than the technical, Tibbits was hesitant in discussing dosages of electrotherapy in other than phenomenalist terms. Like clocks and watches, galvanometers were liable to get out of order. For Tibbits, facts as experienced by the body need not be reconstructed according to the needs of mathematical analyses. Such a phenomenalist approach, therefore, would have been consonant with the beliefs of many Victorian medical men struggling to come to terms with burgeoning electrical technologies in the latter two decades of the nineteenth century.

Alert to the opportunities of social advancement, Tibbits established the West End Hospital for Diseases of the Nervous System, Welbeck Street, on leaving the National Hospital in 1876. A controversial move was the subsequent founding of a School of Massage and Electricity in connection with the hospital to train nurses and masseurs. Tibbits' manual, based on his electrical and anatomical demonstrations delivered at the school, carried the subversive message that the skills and knowledge of the electrotherapeutist could be easily transferred to medical auxiliaries.[34] Irregular practice using popular devices like the magneto-electric machine was, of course, to be condemned, as was the electrically incompetent surgeon who galvanised a little girl for practically three months without realising that 'a connecting wire in the battery was broken; [and thus] no electricity reached the patient'.[35] Familiarisation with galvanometry would ensure that the student would at least know whether or not the batteries were energised. So even surgeons would understand, Tibbits condescendingly remarked. The precautionary measure of testing the current upon oneself before on the patient, linked with the knowledge of graduated dosages, would at least overcome the worst excesses of self-treatment.

Tibbits was aware of the controversial nature of his advocacy of greater autonomy for ancillary medical personnel. He thus tempered his message, stating that methods of treatment should only be administered when prescribed by medical men under their own supervision – and even then only by nurses thoroughly trained and experienced in such application.[36] But skills learned in the classroom and at the bedside had to be augmented by a sort of metrological morality. For Tibbits, the perfect electrician was 'a woman bland, mild, meek, soothing, peaceable, not rough or severe. A gentlewoman who never applies electricity to a patient without first applying it to herself.'[37] Above all, the electrician should not use galvanometry as a screen behind which to cloak her ignorance, just as certain destitute medical electricians found 'refuge' in certain words like 'hysteria.'[38]

The milliampere represented an unnecessary degree of

abstraction in electrotherapeutic practice, Tibbits asserted.[39] 'You are guided entirely not by cells or batteries, but by the position of the needle.' Yet galvanometry could give an accurate estimation of a battery's strength, and Tibbits admitted that this multiplied by the length of time during which the current was applied; doses could thus be meted out. Though deployment of milliamperes was a mere epiphenomenon of the true dosage, electricians had to be prepared to measure milliamperes if asked to do so. The responsibility would then rest upon the doctor, not the electrician. With reluctance, therefore, Tibbits confessed to galvanometric practice. He urged his students to pay only lip service to it – to be cognisant of it, but not to believe in it as a guide to dosage.

The context of Tibbits' reaction to the calls for greater precision in electrotherapy through the use of sophisticated instrumentation had been established by Armand De Watteville, who in the 1870s had argued for a more scientific electrotherapy based on the administration of precise doses of electricity. De Watteville's metrological message, as outlined in his textbook, called for the adoption of the milliampere standard unit of measurement in electrotherapy.[40] 'The milliampere is the most practical unit of measurement. For its multiples correspond to the strength of the currents used in medical applications.'[41] (The British Association's Committee, comprising William Thomson and James Clerk Maxwell, adopted the ohm as a standard of resistance in 1863, though it was not until 1881 that the ampere (named by Helmholtz) was recognised as the unit of current to replace the Weber that had come into use.)

De Watteville's self-styled innovation to adopt the milliampere as a medical unit of current strength to fulfill the goal of metrological precision was, however, mitigated by an awareness that the ampere was a 'constructed' quantity.[42] Compensation for the earth's magnetic field had to be taken into account in order to balance the earth's Oerstedian deflection of a compass needle in the vicinity of a current carrying wire. The earth's magnetic field varied over time and from location to location. De Watteville thus listed in his text the magnetic variations in ten cities over a ten-year period.[43]

With 'Thomsonian' insistence on measurement, De Watteville argued that the intangible world of electrics could be unlocked with instrumentation that manifested concrete realities, based on measurable magnitudes. 'A few days spent in observation with a cell, a rheostat, and a galvanometer, will save many a misunderstanding and make a man a better electrician than as many months reading about Ohm's law and its consequences.'[44] De Watteville clearly did not want his reader to become as attentive to the painstaking detail of electrical measurement as the laboratory physicist. Nevertheless, he insisted that his reader acquire a veneer of the culture of the physicist by providing details on how the medical electrician could calibrate his own galvanometer. Such invocations of Smilesian 'self-help' ensured the integrity of a measurement derived from the procedures and skills of the electrotherapeutician alone.[45] With metrological precision assured, De Watteville thus compared the galvanometer to the scales and weights of the pharmacist. Just as grains of potassium iodide could be administered precisely, so could milliamperes of electricity.[46] However, as with pharmaceutical preparations, De Watteville acknowledged that exogenous factors could stigmatise electrotherapy with the same degree of imprecision. Just as a dose of potassium iodide was affected, for example, by the degree of dilution of the fluids in the body and its rates of elimination, so the size of the electrodes, their relative position and the depth and surroundings of the targeted organ affected the dose. Whether 10, 40 or 80 grains of iodide was a fair average dose raised a similar question as whether 5, 10 or 20 milliamperes was a proper strength to apply.[47] Physiological idiosyncrasies were not a cause for metrological skepticism, De Watteville insisted. 'Much of our posology is still very much a matter of opinion. The more reason then to bring all the methods into play which, though not eliminating every source of fallacy, assist in bringing to a focus the results of a multifarious experience.[48]

Through the sedulous application of galvanometry, De Watteville constructed an electrotherapeutic posology in the light of general principles of 'electro-physics.' Though the irregularities of the human body as an electrical conductor precluded any guide to the actual properties of the current to be used, a clear understanding of what determines 'the flow of electricity under various conditions' would remove the misconceptions and errors that had dominated electrotherapeutic writings and 'prepare the way for more rational modes of action'.[49] Galvanometric readings varied according to the size of the electrodes, length of time and pressure applied, moisture, location and distance between the electrodes. Only by deploying the galvanometer and rheostat could the student himself fully understand the meaning of the relative resistance of the body as measured at different motor points on its surface.

One final posological consideration that needed to be addressed was the quantity of electricity applied. The amount was a quotient of strength and the time during which it flowed. Whether 1, 10 or 50 milliamps passed for 1,000, 100 or 20 seconds, one amp only would be consumed. The crucial question was whether a weak current applied for a long time was equivalent to a strong one for a short period. From a therapeutic point of view, if the electrolytic effects of the current alone were to be taken into account, this would certainly be the case De Watteville asserted. However, if the 'physiological' effects were considered, not only were there limits to the tissues' excitability, but also to the effects of weak and strong excitations which were frequently different or opposite.[50] Posological questions thus simultaneously raised complex issues of therapeutic effect that could not be solved on '*a priori* views,' but 'only upon the data of clinical experience'.[51]

Whereas De Watteville directed his metrological message primarily towards the medical profession, William Stone had the electrical engineer in mind when he came to the rather startling conclusion, after a series of electrical observations on patients in St Thomas's Hospital, that man, electrically speaking, was an 'ambulatory submarine cable'. Using his 1869 Introductory Address to St. Thomas's Hospital as a platform to air his views on metrology, Stone drew on his classical education to explain that perceptions needed to be tested and revised if error was to be avoided in scientific reasoning. Just as astronomers used personal error in their tables and soldiers learned 'judging distance drill', medical students should similarly be taught in the training of the eye, ear and hand.[52] Moreover, the cultivation of the senses and the pursuit of precision, Stone declared, would act as a breakwater against the flood of credulity based on 'flabby beliefs' and 'moral intoxication' that had been engendered by 'the successive shocks men's minds have received from the whirlwind progress of modern science' including the railway, the electric telegraph, photography, and spectroanalysis – which had been exploited by those 'very small magicians, the spirit rappers and table turners'.[53]

Stone experimented on a number of patients at St Thomas's Hospital in the 1880s, and came to the rather novel conclusion that the body acted more in accordance with a solid conductor than a fluid one. Stone had become convinced that there was a relationship between the temperature of the body and its electrical resistance.[54] Furthermore, clinical evidence suggested that, in electrical terms, man was but a 'small ambulatory Atlantic cable'.[55] At the Southport meeting of the British Association in 1883, he presented a partial summary of these findings:[56] (1) electrical resistance had been discovered to vary in disease;[57] (2) in degenerative changes in which fat replaced muscle, resistance increased; (3) in infantile paralysis, the resistance of the paralysed leg was lower than that of the sound leg.

Patients in hospital wards presented their own peculiar experimental conditions with which Stone had to contend: 'The hospital ward is an awkward place for Wheatstone's bridge and delicate galvanometers'.[58] The co-operation of nursing staff was essential. Stone gratefully acknowledged 'the intelligent and kind lady nurses of our hospital ... who ... seconded me in the most self-sacrificing way... to get ready certain patients for me each morning'.[59] Stone favoured large lead and sea water or copper and sea water bucket electrodes in which his patients dipped their feet or hands. The object was to reduce the skin resistance to a minimum. To assist in this aim, the patient's extremities were macerated in saline for periods of half an hour or more. Such a method led Stone to the controversial conclusion that skin resistance had been hitherto over-estimated. On one terminally ill patient Stone obtained 'excellent observations with reversed currents and found them both exactly alike at 1,150 ohms'.[60] After death, Stone inserted two silver needles to a depth of three inches into the plantar muscles of each foot of the corpse. An enormous reduction of resistance was anticipated. However, 'to my surprise the Wheatstone bridge gave 1,200 ohms in either direction of current, or 50 more than with the large lead and salt water electrodes'.[61] The greater resistance was simply due to the added human tissue that the current had to pass through. The skin resistance had thus effectively been reduced to a minimum, or nil.

Further attempts to measure the electrical resistance of the human body using different currents and instruments revealed resistances of 600 and 1,000 ohms, and 1,007 to 1,009 ohms. Two opposite sources of error seemed to be at play; Stone observed a condensed action spuriously lowering the reading with alternating currents, and a polarisation fallaciously raising it with the continuous currents. 'It struck me', Stone concluded, 'that the human body besides being an imperfect conductor resembles a very leaky condenser – in fact it has three attributes – it is a conductor, a condenser and an electrolyte, and it is not dissimilar to a faulty submarine cable'.[62]

At the turn of the century, electromedical technology and metaphor reached its ultimate expression in the work of A. E. Baines (fl. 1860), a submarine cable engineer turned medical enthusiast. Extrapolating from Stone's work, and deploying Kelvin's astatic galvanometer, Baines devised an electropathology based on 'nerve leaks' and proprietary treatments based on 'dielectric oils'.[63] During World War I William Bayliss (1860-1924), the University College Professor of General Physiology, discredited the simplistic model of the body as a submarine cable. The body was not full of free electrons but of ions.[64] The gap between research and practice, however, did not necessarily narrow. Irrational times of war demanded irrational methods in medicine. Conciliation of medical theory and practice seemed a luxury to those in the front line trying to alleviate the sufferings of war. Suspension of professional disdain for empiricism enabled doctors to deploy any method that seemed to work. Heterodox and orthodox practitioners were all in the same boat.

Between 1860 and 1920 the perception of medical therapeutics was transformed by certain doctors who systematically deployed electrical technologies in specialist hospitals for nervous diseases and later in electrical departments in general hospitals. By exploiting the prestige of science and the numinous quality of technology, medical electricians translated the protean forces of nature into an emblem of medical modernity. But instrumentation acted as a two-edged sword for medical electricians; as a means of standardising and conforming the individual to the machine, it enabled doctors to deploy the skills and practices of physicists and electrical engineers in the hope of attaining new insights into disease processes plus greater precision in diagnosis and treatment. Claiming that deployment of the galvanometer was no less alien than using an ordinary clock or a carpenter measuring with a two foot rule, supporters argued that the same degree of precision would be attained in electrotherapy as in physiology. All that was required was some practical experience with the tools of the electrical profession. An electrical posology based on more than the mere tablespoons of the apothecary would become a distinct possibility and an opportunity for inventive medical electricians to market their own galvanometers. Claims for a universalistic scientifically based therapy, however, had to be held in abeyance. As De Watteville and Stone discovered, numerical expression of even such fundamental phenomena as resistance was problematic.

The split in the medical electrical community caused by the introduction of precise instrumentation alienated those like Herbert Tibbits and Julius Althaus who held clinical experience morally and professionally superior to technical knowledge. Underlying their metrological unease was the issue of reconstructing the body according to the needs of quantification; they preferred to deploy the analogical power of batteries and electrical circuits rather than their abstract mathematical formulation. William Stone's deployment of instrumentation, on the other hand, served as a rhetorical tool for exposing 'the flabby beliefs' of the credulous, and those 'morally intoxicated' by scientific and technological progress. With the metrological conviction of a telegraph engineer, Stone affirmed that conflicting measurements of human resistivity did not raise questions about the integrity of the observer and his instruments, but revealed real differences of resistance in the body. Only when the electrical parameters of the body were fully understood in terms of physics, not physiology, would a rational treatment be attained. Such positivism was to fall foul of Bayliss' physiological perspective of electrolytes and ions which undermined electrotherapy's rationale.

Notes

1. W.H. Stone and W.J. Kilner, 'On Measurement in the Medical Application of Electricity' *Journal of the Society of Telegraph Engineers and of Electricians XI* (1882), 107–88: 109.
2. A. De Watteville, 'Review of Von Dr. C. W. Müller's Zur Einleitung in die Elektrotherapie (1885),' *Brain* 8 (1885-1886), 106–107: 106.
3. C. Lawrence, 'Incommunicable Knowledge: Science, Technology and the Clinical Art in Britain 1850-1914,' *Journal of Contemporary History* 20 (1985), 503–20.
4. G. Bird and C. Brooke, *The Elements of Natural Philosophy* (London: John Churchill, 1854, 4th edn).
5. W. Grove, *Correlation of Physical Forces* (London: S. Highley 1846). See I. Morus, 'Marketing the Machine: The Construction of Electrotherapeutics as Viable Medicine in Early Victorian England,' *Medical History* 36 (1992), 34–53.
6. See A. Rabinbach, *The Human Motor: Energy, Fatigue and the Origins of Modernity* (New York: Basic Books, 1990).
7. See R. Williams, 'Cultural Origins and Environmental Implications of Large Technology Systems,' *Science in Context* 62 (1993), 377–403, esp. 390.
8. J. H. Warner describes the 'new physiological therapeutics' in *The Therapeutic Perspective: Medical Practice, Knowledge and Identity in America (1820-1885),* (Harvard: Harvard University Press, 1986).
9. R. Cooter, 'Alternative Medicine, Alternative Cosmology,' *Studies in the History of Alternative Medicine* (ed.) R. Cooter (Basingstoke: Macmillan Press, 1988), 76.
10. See H. W. Lobb, *On the Curative Treatment of Paralysis and Neuralgia and other Affections of the Nervous System with the Aid of Galvanism* (London: Hippolyte Baillière, 1859, 2nd ed.), *Passim*, especially 1–9.

11. C. B. Radcliffe, *Proteus: The Unity of Nature* (London: John Churchill, 1850).

12. See for example, C. B. Radcliffe, 'Abstract, Introductory Lecture, Westminster Hospital,' *Lancet* 2 (1857), 349–350: 349.

13. Anon, 'The Measurement of Nerve Force,' *Nature* 76 (1907), 279–280.

14. S. W. Mitchell, 'The Early History of Instrumental Precision in Medicine,' *Transactions of the College of American Physicians and Surgeons* 2 (1891), 159–181.

15. [C. B. Radcliffe], Minutes (H.50), Royal Medical and Chirurgical Society Scientific Committee No. 3 'Of the Value of Electricity as a Remedial Agent' (13 Oct. 1865 – Jan. 1870).

16. *Ibid.* (1866).

17. J. Althaus, 'Report on Modern Medical Electric and Galvanic Instruments and Recent Improvements in Their Application: with Special Regard to the Requirements of the Medical Practitioner,' *British Medical Journal I* (1873), 44–46, 144–146, 344–345, 740–742, 344,

18. J. Dixon Mann, 'Electro-Therapeutics,' *Lancet* 1 (1877), 191–193.

19. *Ibid.*, 193.

20. A. De Watteville, Letter to the Editor, 'On Current Measurements in Electrotherapeutics,' *Lancet* 1 (1877), 448.

21. *Ibid.*

22. H. Tibbits, 'To the Editor of the Lancet,' *Lancet*, 1 (1877), 448.

23. *Ibid.*

24. *Ibid.*

25. J. Dixon-Mann, Letter to the Editor, 'On Current Measurements in Electro-Therapeutics,' *Lancet* 1 (1877), 483.

26. *Ibid.*

27. *Ibid.*

28. *Ibid.*

29. H. Tibbits, Letter to the Editor, 'On the Current Measurements in Electro-Therapeutics,' *Lancet* 1 (1877), 519.

30. *Ibid.*

31. Dixon-Mann, 'On Current Measurements in Electro-Therapeutics,' *Lancet* 1 (1877), 557.

32. *Ibid.*

33. H. Tibbits, *How to Use a Galvanic Battery in Medicine and Surgery* (London: J. & H. Churchill, 1886), 60.

34. H. Tibbits, *Electrical and Anatomical Demonstrations* (London: J. & H. Churchill, 1887).

35. *Ibid.*, 5.
36. *Ibid.*, 2.
37. *Ibid.*, 6.
38. *Ibid.*, 76.
39. *Ibid.*
40. A. De Watteville, *A Practical Introduction to Medical Electricity* (London: H. K. Lewis, 1879).
41. A. De Watteville, *A Practical Introduction to Medical Electricity* (London: H. K. Lewis, 1884, 2nd ed.), 29.
42. Gooday discusses the interpretive distance that existed between the 'real' measure of a current (based on a calculation synthesis of mass strength and time) and the angular deflection of the tangent galvanometer needle in G. N. Gooday, 'The Morals of Energy Metering: Constructing and deconstructing the precision of the Victorian electrical engineers ammeter and voltmeter' in *Values of Precision*, (ed.) N. Wise, (Princeton: Princeton University Press, 1995).
43. De Watteville, *op. cit.* (note 42), 31.
44. *Ibid.*, 32.
45. S. Smiles, *Self-help* (London: John Murray, 1879, new ed.), as discussed in Gooday, *op. Cit.*
46. De Watteville, *op. cit.* (note 42), 32.
47. *Ibid.*
48. *Ibid.*
49. *Ibid.*, 151.
50. *Ibid.*, 153.
51. *Ibid.*
52. W. H. Stone, *Novus Theaetetus or Science and Sense, being the Introductory Address delivered at St. Thomas's Hospital* (London: J. Churchill & Sons, 1869), 6.
53. *Ibid.*, 17.
54. W. H. Stone, 'On the Electrical Resistance of the Human Body,' Abstract of a Paper Read before the British Association at Southport, *St. Thomas's Hospital Reports* XII (1883), 1–11, 203–213: 5.
55. The journal *Nature* recorded Stone's clinical investigations in a series of 'Notes': W. H. Stone, 'Note on the Influence of High Temperature on the Electrical Resistance of the Human Body,' *Nature* 28 (1883-1884), 151–152, 463–464; 30 (1884), 56, 269–270.
56. Stone, *op. cit.* (note 54), 5.
57. W. H. Stone, 'On Measurement in the Medical Application of

Electricity,' *Journal of the Society of Telegraph Engineers and Electricians* XI (1882), 107–118, 113.

58. Stone, *op. cit.* (note 54), (Abstract, BA Meeting), 208.

59. *Ibid.*, 212.

60. *Ibid.*

61. *Ibid.*

62. W. H. Stone, 'Mance's Method of Eliminating Polarisation: its employment for testing the resistance of the human body,' *The Electrician* XV–XVI (1885-1886), 353–354: 354.

63. A. E. Baines and F. H. Bowman, *Electropathology and Therapeutics, together with a prefaratory treatise on the nervous system and its relation to neuroelectricity by F. H. Bowman* (London: Ewart, Seymour & Co, 1913), 40.

64. W. M. Bayliss, 'The Electrician as Physiologist,' (Review of Studies in Electrophysiology, Animal and Vegetable by Arthur E. Baines), *British Medical Journal* 2 (1918), 160–161: 161.

5

The Introduction of Mathematical Statistics into Medical Research:
The Roles of Karl Pearson, Major Greenwood and Austin Bradford Hill

Eileen Magnello

I look upon statistics as the handmaid of medicine, but on that
very account I hold that it befits medicine to treat her handmaid
with proper respect, and not to prostitute her services for
controversial or personal purposes.[1]

Karl Pearson

This chapter will examine Karl Pearson's role in the medical
community and, in particular, the promulgation of his statistical
methods by his students including Major Greenwood, John Brownlee
and Austin Bradford Hill. Their collective efforts led to the successful
adoption of mathematical statistics in medicine and thereby
transformed medical research in the twentieth century. The value of
mathematical statistics to medical research, they maintained, was that
it provided a set of rigorous tools for workers in clinical or preventive
medicine who were often unable to conduct experiments or who had
to work with records already available (unlike the laboratory worker
who had an already existing set of tools). Medical practitioners argued
that statistical methods could provide 'clearer insight into the
phenomenon of epidemic disease', measure the statistical accuracy of
various instruments, give a 'rational prognosis' and 'secure a logical
basis' for medical research.[2] In short, research undertaken would be
more reliable and the results would afford greater confidence when
appropriate statistical methods were utilised.

Whilst applications of some types of statistics to problems of
biology had been made by Adolphe Quetelet, Francis Galton and
W.F.R. Weldon by the end of the nineteenth century, Pearson
ultimately created a new discipline of mathematical statistics. He did
this when he established the Biometric School in 1893 (and later the

95

Drapers' Biometric Laboratory in 1903), founded the journal *Biometrika* with Weldon and Galton in 1900 and set up the first degree course in statistics in Britain in 1917. Prior to Pearson establishing this new discipline, the General Register's Office had been the centre for the collection and tabulation of medical statistics. The principal form of statistics used throughout much of Victorian Britain was, in fact, vital statistics and actuarial methods. This use and type of statistics began to change in the 1870s when Francis Galton began to examine statistical and biological variation and showed that standardised comparisons could be made by using the law of frequency (or the normal distribution).

At the end of the nineteenth century, the content and practice of statistics underwent a series of transitions that led to its emergence as a highly specialised mathematical discipline. These intellectual (and later institutional) changes were, in part, brought about by a mathematical-statistical translation of the Darwinian change in ideas about what kinds of natural processes occur in the world. The Darwinian idea that had the greatest impact on the development of mathematical statistics, was Darwin's redefinition of the biological species as something which could be viewed in terms of populations; in contrast, the Aristotelian essentialistic idea of 'types', which formed the basis of the morphological or typological concept of species used by a number of biologists until the end of the 19th century, focused on averages rather than on individual variation. Pearson's and Weldon's mathematical reconceptualisation of Darwinian 'statistical' populations of species in the 1890s, thus provided the framework within which a major paradigmatic shift occurred in statistical techniques and theory.[3] This view is, however, in contrast to much of the scholarship on the origins of Pearsonian statistics. Most historians have argued that Pearson's interests in eugenics provided the impetus to the development of his statistics.[4] This argument has, however, not only overlooked Pearson's earliest statistical work, but it has also neglected the totality and complexity of the full range of the various quantitative and statistical methods that Pearson devised and deployed in all four of his laboratories.[5]

Vital statistics

Hence, two different statistical methodologies were created in the nineteenth century which differed ideologically, conceptually and mathematically and these distinctions may be seen in Figure 5.1. Vital statistics, which is undoubtedly the way in which the word 'statistics' is most commonly understood, is used as a plural noun as

Fig.5.1
'Differences between vital statistics and mathematical statistics'

VITAL STATISTICS		MATHEMATICAL STATISTICS
	FORM:	
ENUMERATIVE		ANALYTICAL
PLURAL NOUN		SINGULAR NOUN
(Data, Censuses,		(corpus of statistical methods
General Records Office)		underpinned by theoretical-
		mathematical infrastructure)
	IDEOLOGY:	
ARISTOTELIAN		DARWINIAN
ESSENTIALISM		POPULATION OF SPECIES
	MEASURES:	
AVERAGES	and	VARIATION
(mean, median, mode)		(standard deviation, coefficient of
		variation, standard error of
		estimate)
	METHODS:	
		Correlational techniques:
		1. parametric and non-parametric
Census counts		*2. simple and multiple*
Life Tables		*3. independent and matched samples*
Percentages		The chi-square goodness of fit
Ratios		test and chi-square test of association
Proportions		The Design of Experiments
Student's t-test		(e.g., the Analysis of Variance)
	PROBABILITY:	
Actuarial Methods		Significance Tests
	STATISTICIANS:	
FRANCIS BISSET HAWKINS		KARL PEARSON
ADOLPHE QUETELET		GEORGE UDNY YULE
SOUTHWOOD SMITH		W. S. GOSSET ['STUDENT']
PIERRE LOUIS	FRANCIS GALTON	MAJOR GREENWOOD
WILLIAM AUGUSTUS GUY		JOHN BROWNLEE
WILLIAM FARR		PERCY STOCKS
FLORENCE NIGHTINGALE		RAYMOND PEARL
EDWIN CHADWICK		RONALD A. FISHER
RONALD ROSS		AUSTIN BRADFORD HILL
	MEDICAL ISSUES:	
EPIDEMIOLOGY		"INHERITANCE OF DISEASE"
PUBLIC HEALTH		(e.g., Tuberculosis, cancer)
SANITARY REFORMS		EPIDEMIOLOGY
		CLINICAL MEDICINE
		THERAPEUTIC TRIALS

97

it refers to an aggregate set of data, and could be best described as an enumerative process as would be employed in census counts or in the tabulation of vital and official statistics. This would include, for example, crime statistics, divorce statistics and cricket statistics all of which were used throughout the nineteenth century and continue to be used in the twentieth century. Vital statistics is quite often concerned with the measurement of averages and, ideologically, much of its use is underpinned by Aristotelian essentialism such as that espoused by Quetelet. The principal tools used include life tables, averages, percentages, proportions and ratios: probability is used most commonly for actuarial purposes.

The medical issues that nineteenth century statisticians addressed most typically included epidemiology, public health and sanitary reforms. (Whilst epidemiology was a concern to vital statistics, it would continue to play a central role in the newly created discipline of mathematical statistics.) Some of the better known medical statisticians who fall under the rubric of vital statistics include Francis Bisset Hawkins (1796-1894) whose book, *The Elements of Medical Statistics,* was published in 1829.[6] Hawkins defined medical statistics as 'the application of numbers to illustrate the natural history of man in health and disease [which gave] the most convincing proofs of the efficacy of medicine'.[7] *The Elements* was a compendium of vital data taken from a variety of late eighteenth and early nineteenth century published sources. The book was 'illustrative of the comparative salubrity, longevity, mortality, and prevalence of diseases in the principal countries and cities of the civilised world'. Moreover, statistics was considered to be one of the 'easiest arguments that can be employed to refute the vulgar notion ... that nature is alone sufficient for the cure of disease'.[8] Thomas Southwood Smith (1788-1861) collected statistical data in 1837 'on the physical causes of sickness and mortality to which the poor are particularly exposed'. Born in the same year as Hawkins, was the Belgium astronomer and statistician, Adolphe Quetelet (1796-1874) who influenced the use and development of statistics in Britain during this time.

Two years after the Civil Registration Act of 1837, the archetypal mid-Victorian statistician, William Farr (1807-1883) was appointed Compiler of Abstracts to the Registrar General because he was considered to be 'the only medical man who paid any attention to vital statistics'.[9] This material enabled Farr to develop a comprehensive nosology which listed secondary and tertiary causes of death; this was of much benefit not only to the medical profession, but to the assurance societies as well. Farr subsequently founded the

British Annals of Medicine in 1837 which was the first medical journal to use vital statistics. A year later the *BMJ* and the *Lancet* were providing monthly reports on the vital statistics of Britain as well as of foreign countries. John Eyler regarded Farr as 'the first person to adequately describe an epidemic numerically' by extending the actuary's technique of discovering the law of mortality in a life table.[10]

In 1859, the medically trained statistician, William Augustus Guy (1810-1888) delivered the Croonian Lecture at the Royal College of Physicians on 'The Numerical Method and its Application to the Science and Art of Medicine'.[11] Guy argued that studies of human disease and health were 'a source of difficulty and complexity' owing to the vast amount of differences in humans. When looking at hundreds of cases, the numerical method (which quite often meant 'averages'), could help to make data more manageable and thus help to illuminate their conditions. Guy also took an active role in the Statistical Society of London and was its President from 1873-187.

Florence Nightingale and the Chair of Applied Statistics

Many of the early papers published in the *Statistical Society Journal* were, in fact, written by members of the medical profession which included reports on disease, illness, mortality and hospital conditions. With regards to hospital statistics, an important figure involved in this statistical movement is Florence Nightingale (1820-1910). Known primarily for her role as a nurse in the Crimean War, Nightingale who has often been described as a 'passionate statistician', regarded statistics as 'the most important science in the world'. Statistics also took on a spiritual element for Nightingale as she maintained that 'to understand God's thoughts, we must study statistics for these are the measure of His purpose'.[12] She shared with Francis Galton the idea that the statistical study of natural phenomena was 'the religious duty of man'.[13] Her statistical work was influenced by Farr, Galton and Quetelet, and she was elected a fellow of the Statistical Society of London in 1858.

A year later, Nightingale realised that various London hospitals (including St. Thomas', St. Bartholomew's and University College London) were using their own system of naming and classifying disease, and it was not possible to compare mortality rates or different diseases among patients in the various London hospitals. She subsequently embarked on a campaign to establish uniform reporting and the classification of mortality and disease statistics for hospitals. With the assistance of Farr and others, she drew up a standard list of diseases and drafted model hospital statistical forms which would:

99

enable us to ascertain the relative mortality of different hospitals, as well as of different diseases and injuries at the same and different ages, the relative frequency of different disease and injuries among the classes which enter hospitals in different counties, and in different districts of the same counties.[14]

Pearson regarded Nightingale as a very good administrator guided by a knowledge of statistics. She had such a high regard for statistics that in 1891 she wrote to Sir Douglas Galton (a cousin of Francis Galton) that she wanted to establish a Professorship or Readership in Applied Statistics at Oxford. By then she was no longer thinking primarily about the statistics of hygiene and sanitary work 'because these and their statistics have been more closely studied in England than probably any other branch of statistics'.[15] She was, for example, interested in undertaking a statistical study of the utility of education after children leave school and determining whether all 'they have been taught is *waste*'.[16] When Pearson read Nightingale's letter to Sir Douglas Galton he thought that it was 'the finest letter she ever wrote' and that ' the prophetess was proclaiming my own creed'.[17]

She discussed her plan of setting up the Professorship with Francis Galton who thought that it would be more suitable to train applied statisticians by six lectures a year at the Royal Institution. Pearson thought that Nightingale had the better scheme: although the 'Royal Institution was valuable for announcing in a popular way the results of recent research, it was not an academic centre for training enthusiastic young minds to a new department in science'.[18] Pearson held that Nightingale's desire to create such a Chair should somehow be commemorated; thus, some twenty years later, when he was looking for a new name for his newly established department, he thought that 'no fitter and worthy name occurred to me than that of "Applied Statistics"'.[19]

Galtonian versus Pearsonian statistics

The person who serves as the bridge between the medical-vital statistics of mid-Victorian Britain and the mathematical statistics of Karl Pearson is Francis Galton (1822-1911) who was a medical student at Birmingham in 1838. Two years after he had begun his studies, he went up to Cambridge to take a degree in mathematics. At this time Galton thought that 'mathematics would be beneficial in his later career as a Doctor'. However, he gave up his medical studies after he inherited his father's money and managed eventually to get a Third class in the mathematics tripos at Cambridge. With this aforementioned group of vital statisticians, Galton shared the idea that statistics could be used to enumerate social conditions, but he differed from this group because he was *also* interested in measuring the biological variation (elucidated by his half-cousin Charles Darwin) for which he devised some statistical methods. Galton, however, retained an essentialistic outlook with respect to both statistics and biological species and thus he does not fit neatly into either group.

The link to Pearson is that Galton devised graphical measures of simple correlation and simple regression. Whilst Galton endorsed the idea of Pearson's statistical innovations, he never used any of Pearson's methods: they differed fundamentally in their use of the normal distribution. Galton was convinced that all biological data should conform to the normal distribution (i.e., the symmetric bell-shaped curve) – as if to say that all biological data were static. Pearson, however, recognised that biological data varied and did not conform to the normal distribution. Hence this variation meant that distributions of biological data could take on a variety of different shapes (which included, for example, symmetric, asymmetric, J-shaped or U-shaped distributions). Pearson's detection of the asymmetry in biological data provided the linchpin to the construction of his mathematical statistics. Over a period of seven years Pearson's statistical innovations led to a divergence from vital statistics when he established the following procedures:

1. In 1893 he introduced the standard deviation which could be used to measure variation at all points on the distribution; vital statistical methods instead measured averages using such procedures as the mean, median and mode.
2. He made statistics a much more mathematically rigorous discipline when he introduced matrix algebra into statistics in 1896.[20]
3. When he devised the chi-square goodness of fit test in 1900 and used the chi-square distribution, he provided a procedure for determining the level of statistical significance between two variables.[21]

Like Galton, Pearson went up to Cambridge to read mathematics, but unlike Galton, Pearson found that the highly competitive and demanding system leading up to the mathematical tripos was the tonic he needed – since he had been a rather delicate and sickly child with a nervous disposition. Once at Cambridge his health improved, whereas much the opposite happened to Galton.[22] Pearson graduated with honours being Third Wrangler in 1879.

Having started his career as an elastician (that is, someone who derived mathematical equations for elastic properties of matter), Pearson pursued a number of areas before he settled on mathematical statistics. Shortly after finishing the Mathematical Tripos examination, he decided to read philosophy at Cambridge in preparation for his trip to Germany. After making arrangements with Kuno Fischer, he left for Heidelberg on 14 April 1879 to ' improve his German and to study physics and metaphysics' with Fischer, Kirchoff and Helmholtz. Soon afterwards, and much to his chagrin, he realised that he 'would never be a great mathematician or physicist like [James] Clerk Maxwell, [William] Thomson or [Hermann von] Helmholtz'. He discovered next that as 'philosophy made him miserable', he wasn't going to be a great philosopher either. He then decided to study Roman Law in Berlin. However, by the beginning of 1880, he was 'tired of the law' and thought instead that it was 'perhaps time [he] fell in love'. Nevertheless, he was called to the Bar at the end of 1881 which, in his limited experience, he found a rather depressing practice.[23]

Having decided that he 'shall have no more law', he decided 'to devote [his] time to the religious producing of German literature before 1300'. Though he was short-listed for a newly created post in German at Cambridge in the summer of 1884,[24] he 'longed to be working with symbols and not words'.[25] After having been rejected from more than six mathematical posts over a period of two years, he received the Chair of 'Mechanism and Applied Mathematics' at UCL in the autumn of 1884 and he began teaching mathematical physics to engineering students. Soon after he also gave lectures in astronomy and helped students with research work on graphics for the Engineering Degree.[26]

In 1890 he took up another post in the Gresham Chair of Geometry which he held for three years concurrently with his post at UCL. His Gresham Lectures signified a turning-point in Pearson's career and owing, in particular, to his relationship with W.F.R. Weldon who was the first biologist Pearson met who was interested in using a statistical approach for problems of Darwinian evolution.[27] Their emphasis on Darwinian population of species, not only implied the necessity of systematically measuring variation, but it prompted the re-conceptualisation of statistical populations for Pearson and Weldon. It was this mathematisation of Darwin that led to a paradigmatic shift for Pearson from the Aristotelian essentialism underpinning vital statistics. Weldon's questions provided the impetus for Pearson's seminal statistical work which led eventually to the creation of the Biometric School at UCL in October 1894. Hence, began a lifelong interest in applying statistical methods to problems of biology and also to medicine. Some of the methods that Pearson devised to measure variation and correlation are listed in Figure 1. (Pearson devised at least 18 methods of correlation and he also devised both chi-square tests.)[28] Since Pearson had no formal training in biology or in medicine, he relied on people like Weldon and Major Greenwood to assist him in these matters.

Family pedigrees and the inheritance of disease

Pearson's first successful attempt to engage the medical profession in some sort of quantitative work was through the collection of hundreds and thousands of pieces of pathological data for the construction of more than one thousand family pedigrees. His family pedigrees, which were assembled in an attempt to discover the inheritance of various diseases included such conditions as diabetes, paralysis, alcoholism, insanity, epilepsy, pulmonary tuberculosis and cancer. The significance of these pedigrees is twofold: firstly, the medical doctors who assisted Pearson began systematically to collect a greater amount of data than they had done previously and assembled it in a coherent and meaningful arrangement, and secondly, the collection of this data and the construction of these family pedigrees enabled these doctors to move away from concentrating on individual pathological cases or 'types' and to see, instead, a wide range of pathological variation of any number of diseases (or conditions). Hence, the ideological move from Aristotelian essentialism to the variation underpinning statistical populations. There was, admittedly, a mixed response from the medical community: some doctors thought the collection of family pedigrees 'should be an essential part of their work'[29] whereas others thought 'medical men would be fools to give any help to any biometrician'.[30]

When Pearson decided with 'much reluctance' to take over the Eugenics Record Office (which he renamed the Eugenics Laboratory at the end of 1906),[31] he wrote to Galton that:

> I want to make the Eugenics Laboratory a centre for information and inquiry. I want to extend the tendency which is growing up outside for social and medical workers to send their observations to the Biometric Laboratory. But to do this, I think we ought to try and associate half dozen [medical] men to the Laboratory as an advisory committee or as associates.[32]

He suggested the following: Dr John Macpherson, the Lunacy Commissioner in Scotland, Lieutenant Colonel William Simpson in the Royal Army Medical Department; the actuarialist, William Palin Elderton, Dr Mott who worked on the inheritance of lunacy and Edward Nettleship, the ophthalmic surgeon. Pearson proposed at once to issue definite disease pedigree schedules for children whose family had a history of alcohol, cancer, paralysis, insanity, epilepsy, or tuberculosis. By then David Heron, medical officer in the Eugenics Laboratory, had collected 400 cases for an insanity pedigree and Pearson had gathered more than 400 cases for tuberculosis. From February 1908 to June 1909, John Bulloch of the London Hospital Medical College collected data for family pedigrees on diabetes and tuberculosis, and Dr T Lewis of UCH Medical College, provided data for the inheritance of polydactyly, brachydactyly and split-foot.

Pearson adopted many of the techniques and resources from the vital statistics of the General Register's Office (GRO) in the Eugenics Laboratory. Galton had also advocated using actuarial methods for problems of eugenics which Pearson utilised when he became the Director of this Laboratory in 1907. He also used mortality rates from the GRO when comparing national death rates to local death rates for certain diseases such as TB and cancer. Though Pearson used five of his more than 25 biometric methods as ancillary measures for problems of eugenics, his principal methodology of actuarial methods was developed out of vital statistics. His family pedigrees served as another quantitative tool for this work. (See Figure 5.2 for an example of one of his pedigrees for degeneracy.)[33]

By 1911 Pearson was receiving assistance from more than 16 medical doctors (including Major Greenwood) from various London hospitals. These doctors were engaged in the collection of hundreds and sometimes thousands of cases that could be used to construct family pedigrees. Some of the other doctors included Sir James Crichton-Browne who sent Pearson elaborate measurements of the brains of 400 insane individuals and Dr R. Langdon Down who had given the Laboratory notes on over 2,000 cases of idiocy. Pearson also attended meetings of the Royal Society of Medicine quite regularly to ask various medical practitioners for data for his pedigrees. Virtually all of this material was published in a thesaurus of family pedigrees of pathological, physical and mental data in the collected works of the *Treasury of Family Inheritance* (the first volume was published in March 1909 and the last in 1930). The *Treasury* thus represented Pearson's first attempts to encourage doctors to see that certain kinds of medical data could be quantified systematically.

The statistics of anti-typhoid vaccinations and tuberculosis

Pearson's desire to apply his statistical methods to medicine was most evident in the first two decades of the twentieth century. By then, he

Fig. 5.2
Pedigrees for Cataract and Degeneracy

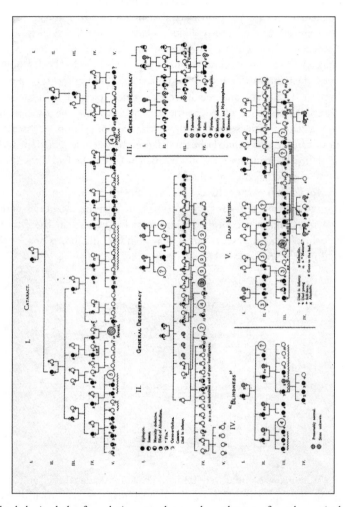

had devised the foundations to the modern theory of mathematical statistics. During this time he became engaged in a series of debates in the *BMJ*, the *Lancet* and the *Journal of the Royal Society of Medicine* on various statistical matters relating to tuberculosis, insanity, alcoholism and anti-typhoid vaccinations.

The first of these debates was on the efficacy of anti-typhoid vaccinations. In 1896 the bacteriologist, Almroth Wright (1861-1947) developed a vaccine to protect against typhoid. Since he worked in the Royal Army Medical College, Wright used his vaccine on soldiers in transit to India. Due to some disputes the War Office had with Wright, they wanted to assess the statistical reliability of these results. Lieutenant Colonel Simpson asked Pearson for his advice and gave him two sets of data of anti-typhoid inoculation statistics which were divided into two groups. The first group consisted of regiments in South Africa and the second was from regiments in India. Both groups were then sub-divided into two classes of mortality experience (recovered or died) and incidence experience (escaped or infected). Pearson then wanted to reduce the data by measuring the association of inoculation with escape (i.e., those who did not develop the disease) and then he determined the association between inoculation and mortality. He computed the phi coefficient (which he had devised in 1900) and averaged these values.[34]

To compute the phi coefficient, the frequency surface of a normal distribution was divided into four separate categories with two rows and two columns.[35] The total frequencies in these four categories were represented by *a, b, c, d,* in four quadrants of a four-fold table. (See Table 5.1)

Table 5.1
Mortality Experience

	Recovered	Died	
Escaped	a	b	
			Incidence
Infected	c	t	

When *a, b, c,* and *d* were known, Pearson calculated the values by using the ordinary table of the probability integral provided by William Fleetwood Sheppard.[36] An association could be found only if groupings had been made into the four groups a, b, c, and d using the formula:

$$r_{hk} = \frac{ad - bc}{\sqrt{(b + d)(a + c)(c + d)(a + b)}}$$

The values of association that Pearson calculated from this data ranged from 0.12 to 0.45, and most of the there were quite low (i.e., less than 0.30).[37] When Pearson averaged these values, the correlation was 0.23, and such a low value cast 'doubt on whether this [was] sufficiently large to identify the treatment being adopted as routine'.[38] Pearson thus concluded that the average correlation was too low to warrant the use of the anti-typhoid vaccination, and the *BMJ* supported Pearson's conclusions.[39] In addition to its analytic conclusions for medical practice, this short paper contained two seminal statistical ideas. First, Pearson suggested a clinical trial of sorts (using alternate people as a control group) and secondly, his procedure of averaging the phi-coefficient represents one of the earliest uses of what statisticians today would term 'meta-analysis'.[40]

A year after this debate with Wright, Pearson became involved in the debates on the use of sanatoriums for treatment of pulmonary tuberculosis and wrote more than 20 letters to the *BMJ*. Before 1880 there was an overriding view that tuberculosis was the product of hereditary diathesis or constitution, 'whereby the presence of tubercles was a consequence of disease rather than its cause'.[41] Pearson thought that 'the diathesis of tuberculosis is certainly inherited, and the intensity of the inheritance is sensibly the same as that of any normal physical character yet investigated in Man'.[42] He also found that the elder offspring in a family appeared more likely to become subject to tuberculosis than other family members.

In the midst of one of these debates occurs Pearson's earliest discussion on the use of random sampling. Rather than using case-notes from one doctor only, he suggested the following procedures to construct a random sample of the general population for whom the absolute presence or absence of a disease (such as tuberculosis or cancer) has been determined:

1. Ascertain the prevalence of the disease or character in the population at large by using mortality statistics, or more exactly from combined medical experience.

2. Take a sample of 1,000 persons with the disease and record the incidence of the disease among their ancestry and collaterals. (This can be done from casebooks of the specialist.)

3. Take a sample of 1,000 persons without the special disease and investigate the distribution of the disease among their ancestry and collaterals from special inquiry or information from casebooks from GPs.[43]

Pearson claimed to have had no medical opinion on the use of sanatoriums for TB. His family pedigrees seem to have suggested to him that tuberculosis was inherited, and he also thought that natural selection was affecting the mortality rate for patients who had TB. In an attempt to tackle the problems of tuberculosis, he had envisaged a 'co-operative effort of medical specialist, general practitioner and statisticians'. He then asked 'is it not time that some organisation be created for collecting in bulk and reducing medical statistics bearing on inheritance?'[44] Pearson looked upon statistics as the 'handmaid of medicine', but he also held that medicine should 'treat her handmaid with proper respect, and not to prostitute her services for controversial or personal purposes'.[45]

He went on to say that whilst he was 'not concerned with the medical side' of the sanatorium treatment of tuberculosis, he was, however, 'concerned with the statistical evidence by means of which the contrast between pre-sanatorium treatment and modern treatment has been established by Dr. Latham and Mr Garland in their book on *The Conquest of Consumption*'. Pearson explained that they took data from Dr Pollock's book *The Elements of Prognosis in Consumption* (1865), where Pollock had shown 'that 83% of his patients were alive after five years'. Since Latham and Garland wanted to show, however, the 'grim state of affairs in pre-sanatorium days' they converted Pollock's patients into 'dead men'.[46] Pearson went on to say that 'this is a very grave matter indeed'. Thus, he concluded that 'my aim is not to attack inconclusive results, but to induce investigators to adopt better methods'.[47]

Five days after Pearson's letter appeared in the *BMJ*, he wrote to Greenwood that he had received

> quite a number of good letters, including one from Sir James Barr, about the Latham-Garland business, and it is quite a pleasure to feel that there are a number of medical men who realise that some stop has got to be put to the wild statements of the medical advertisers.[48]

Barr wrote to Pearson after reading one of his papers on multiple correlation and to say that

> I believe that all problems will eventually have to be settled by statistics, but to my mind the process is too slow. It is always wise to survey our position and see whether we are progressing in the right line. Statistics will show us whether we are right or wrong, but if wrong, the cry of halt will not show us what other course we should adapt. We must then fall back on experience.[49]

Two weeks later, William Paget-Tomlinson and John Guy wrote to the *BMJ* providing tables containing data for the number of patients who had tuberculosis, the number of years in treatment at a sanatorium and the outcome of the treatment (e.g. quite well, fair, frail, dead and untraced).[50] Paget-Tomlinson had opened one of the first sanatoria in Britain when he established the Westmorland Sanatorium for Consumption near Grange-over-Sands in 1900, with accommodation for 16 patients. By 1910 he had room for 60 beds and was looking to open another institution for 25 'advanced cases'.[51] He maintained that 'any sanatorium which does not report progress of cases for some years after discharge is guilty of a serious omission, and naturally lays itself open to grave criticism'.[52] Guy was 'becoming more and more convinced that the value of the sanatorium is not curative, but educative'.[53]

Pearson replied to the BMS that the valuable letters of:

> Dr Paget-Tomlinson and Dr John Guy in your last issue tend to emphasise the very points I have at heart and which I am quite sure the medical profession also have at heart. We all want to find an exact measurement of the improvement introduced by sanatorium treatment. There is only one way in which this can be done, namely, by measuring in a scientific manner the number of patients exposed to risk and the number that die within the years that they have been exposed to risk.[54]

Pearson used actuarial cards for entering information rapidly about TB and other diseases or medical conditions which he then handed over to the actuary, William Palin Elderton (who had worked in Pearson's Biometric Laboratory). Pearson suggested that other medical men could use actuarial cards and he maintained that it was 'the professional and highly trained actuary who could help to determine the efficacy of sanatorium treatment'.[55]

Several weeks later, Pearson again emphasised the statistician's view that 'to compare the mortality in pre-sanatorium and post-sanatorium days we must have statistics of all types of cases'.[56] He did not suggest this 'in any spirit of aggressive criticism, but to indicate how difficult it is to pronounce a real judgement in the matter until the statistical side is fully appreciated'.[57] He further cautioned that with only a partial knowledge of the recorded cases, where as much as 77% of the data could be missing due to unrecorded cases, and sometimes ' recorded cases disappear from the record', such that 'no definite judgement can be made of sanatorium treatment from the actuarial standpoint'.[58] It seemed to Pearson that what was needed was 'rather the presentation of statistical material relating to heredity and relating to mortality'.[59] Moreover, the contributions of Dr Paget-Tomlinson and Dr Guy had indicated to Pearson that 'the case for sanatoriums as based on lessened mortality is not proven'.[60]

The promotion of statistics

Pearson wrote letters regularly to the *Lancet,* the *BMJ* and the *Journal of the Royal Society of Medicine*. These three journals published well over 50 letters and notes from Pearson as well as reviews of his books and pamphlets. The great bulk of these letters appear between 1900 to 1920. During this time, when Pearson was encouraging or insisting that the medical profession should incorporate rigorous mathematical statistics for medical research, a considerable amount of rhetoric was generated on the use of medical statistics. Thus, for example, in 1900 Philip Henry Pye-Smith delivered a paper on 'Medicine as a Science and Medicine as an Art' at the Annual Meeting of the BMA at Ipswich and he argued that 'rational progress rests on the science of statistics'.[61] There were, however, no suggestions as to how the 'science of statistics' could be put into practice.

Seven years later the editor of the *BMJ* wrote: 'it has long been known than many of the problems with which the medical profession has to deal can only be solved by an application of statistical processes...[and] thanks to the work of Karl Pearson and his pupils (in the last 15 years) it can be said that his school transformed statistics into a branch of exact science'.[62] He stressed, however, that 'it [was] undesirable that we should have in the future two classes of investigators – statisticians who know little of medicine and medical men who know nothing of statistics'.[63] In 1910 the *Lancet* gave a more detailed and somewhat more technical account of Pearsonian statistics than had appeared in the *BMJ* previously.[64] Its authors, James Troup and Darrell Maynard remarked that 'We know that there is the growing up among medical men that the study of mathematics is playing a more intimate part in medicine than heretofore.'[65] Though a number of medical men recognised the importance of mathematical statistics for medicine, the practice of incorporating statistics into medical research was slow. The *BMJ*, for example, heartily recommended Troup's and Maynard's article

> to the many readers who desire to attain a knowledge of statistical methods sufficient to enable them to follow the numerous technical papers in which these methods are applied to medical and pathological problems.[66]

The *BMJ* had often expressed the opinion that the importance of modern mathematical-statistical discoveries would soon be recognised in the medical world. As evidence of the 'correctness' of their view, they were pleased to announce in 1910 that the governing body of the Lister Institute of Preventive Medicine had appointed Major Greenwood as a whole-time member of their staff and established a statistical department. Though the number of medical men who had received an adequate training in mathematical statistics was still small, the journal noted that it was increasing steadily.[67] Yet when the malariaist, Ronald Ross (1857-1932), began to study mathematically the problems involved in the spread of malaria, the editor of the *BMJ* wrote that:

> Although it will be no news to those who have closely followed Sir Ronald Ross's career, some members of this profession will learn with surprise, possibly mingled with regret, that this distinguished exponent of the experimental method is an enthusiast for the application of quantitative processes to the problems of epidemiology and pathology.[68]

Ronald Ross and 'the problem of the random walk'

In his report on malaria in Mauritius and in the first edition of his treatise on the *Prevention of Malaria,* Ross studied mathematically the problems involved in the spread of malaria.[69] Ross thought that 'all epidemiology, concerned as it is with the variation of diseases from time to time or from place to place *must* be considered mathematically... if it is to be considered scientifically at all'.[70] Though he recognised the importance of measuring variation, he did not have any formal grounding in mathematical-statistics to analyse biological variation.[71] Whilst the *BMJ* was a bit sceptical of Ross's approach, they remarked that 'The medical researcher may not be prepared to go the whole way with Sir Ronald Ross in this statement, but he will be compelled to admit that the methods advocated have to be seriously reckoned with [by] a modern investigator'.[72]

In Ross's first extant letter to Pearson in 1905 he made some mathematical enquires connected with the diffusion of mosquitoes. He wanted to know

> if *n* mosquitoes (or other animals) are liberated at a point and allowed to wander in all directions without special attraction towards one direction, what will be this function giving their numbers at a given moment (e.g., at death) at a distance and from the point? I suppose it is exponential.[73]

Pearson responded with a short note in *Nature* on 'The problem of the random walk'.[74] Ross thanked Pearson for his effort and wrote to him that 'my experiences coincide with yours with regard to the difficulty of getting [doctors to use] pure mathematics to look at a biological subject'.[75] Shortly after this note was published, Pearson and one of his students, John Blakeman, wrote a full paper on Random Migration. In this paper they discussed a problem which arose in attempting to forecast the rate at which a possible habitat would be infiltrated by a species not yet established there. Their work was followed up by John Brownlee in a paper in which he examined the epidemic distributions of the plague in Hong Kong using the mathematical theory of random migration. Brownlee's problem was similar to that suggested by Ross in connection with the spread of mosquitoes within cleared districts.[76]

In some respects, Pearson's attempts to encourage the medical community to adopt more rigorous forms of mathematical statistics (when problems of medical research lent themselves to this sort of analysis), would seem not to have been as successful as he would have hoped. Many of the articles about the importance of using mathematical statistics contained more rhetoric than the actual practice of using statistical methods for medicine. The emphasis on rhetoric and the reluctance to utilise statistics was 'attributed in part to a number of doctors who found mathematics 'obscure and repellent''. It was not only Pearson's statistical methods that were too mathematical for this group; many of the early Mendelians encountered the same problem.[77]

Major Greenwood and medical statistics

It was, however, to the efforts of a number of Pearson's students who taught and promulgated the use of Pearsonian statistics that a transformation in medical research occurred. His first medical student, Major Greenwood, wrote to Pearson in March 1902 about a paper he had been working on concerning the inheritance of moths which he wanted to submit to *Biometrika* (the paper was published 18 months later). Greenwood, who was then a medical student at the London Hospital, wanted to 'begin a quantitative investigation at [Pearson's Biometric] Laboratory on the weights of the spleen, liver, heart and the brain.'[78] In September he came to the Biometric Laboratory to begin this investigation. Two years later he began to work in this laboratory more regularly and continued to work with Pearson for nearly 30 years. After Greenwood decided that he wanted to spend more time in the Biometric Laboratory Pearson cautioned him that:

in the first place if you stick to medical work you should look upon any biometric work you may do as helping to make you intellectually keener, and this increased mental fitness will not be lost in ordinary professional work... It is [nonetheless] very difficult with biometry, there are at present no teaching posts, no demonstratorships or fellowships to aid a young man on his way... If you come to me I will do the best I can to give you a bit of hard work to do.[79]

One of Greenwood's next projects involved the statistics of the opsonic index. (Rosser Matthews discusses this in greater detail in Chapter 6).

When Greenwood was Medical Statistician at the Lister Institute, Pearson mentioned that he wished he 'could get a great Statistical Laboratory with £4,000 per annum increase, and I could ask [William Palin] Elderton, [William Sealy Gosset] 'Student' and you to join hands! There would be plenty of work to do, and the work done would be worth the money to the Nation.'[80] Greenwood replied:

> that we biometricians are looking up, there is not only your own experience but since I have been at the Lister people of really high standing in experimental medicine have submitted results to me for statistical criticism... the time will come and come soon when the just claims of the class of experts, you above all the others have encouraged and trained, are publicly acknowledged just as bacteriologists are recognised.[81]

Greenwood then asked Pearson if 'it would be possible to form a little club, not a society, consisting of you, Elderton, [David] Heron, [John] Bulloch and myself and not more than half a dozen other ... to meet for mutual discussion and criticism of work in medical statistics'.[82] There is, however, no evidence to suggest that the club ever materialised.

At the end of 1922 Greenwood was made Reader in Medical Statistics in the University of London. Around this time Pearson and Greenwood had begun to work on a 'Memorandum on the need for Statistical Training in the Medical Curriculum' so that medical statistics would become a formal requirement for doctors. They wrote that:

> In our opinion the standard of medical education in respect of the large and growing class of medical problems which must be treated upon statistical lines is not only very low but it is calculated to

impair the usefulness and public credit of the medical profession...
we submit that for Post-graduate degrees and diplomas... the
Council should insist upon a knowledge of the elements of
statistics... there is not a single university or licensing body whose
examiners for the diploma of public health would or could reject a
candidate on the ground of his insufficient knowledge of statistical
method.[83]

They remarked that it was often the case that whilst 'a somewhat
high standard of knowledge of bacteriological methods [was] insisted
upon, the test of the knowledge of statistical methods is
perfunctory'.[84] Medical officers of health usually secured the expert
assistance of professional bacteriologists, but were themselves usually
responsible for the compilation, analysis and interpretation of
statistical data. As a result the statistical parts of the health reports
were 'nearly always, extremely superficial, if not actually misleading'.

Pearson and Greenwood hoped that the results of the proposals
would lead ultimately to the creation of a body of medical
statisticians. They argued that such a body was urgently needed not
only for the progress of medical science, but for many purposes of
medical science which included both central and municipal
executives. Several months later (at the beginning of 1923),
Greenwood began to teach a course of 20 lectures on Epidemiology
and Vital Statistics in Pearson's Biometric Laboratory for the Diploma
of Public Health: enforced attendance was recommended by the
General Medical Council.[85] Greenwood taught actuarial methods
from vital statistics as well as Pearson's mathematical statistics.

In the following year, Greenwood delivered a lecture at the
Institute of Pathology at St. Mary's Hospital stressing the importance
of using statistical methods for medical research.[86] In the version of
this paper which appeared in the *Lancet*, he was, nonetheless, quite
careful to express technical ideas in terms that his audience would
understand, and much of the language he adopted was couched in a
relatively non-threatening (i.e., non-mathematical) way. He quite
often did not even name which of Pearson's statistical methods he
used, if anything, he referred to them in a fairly vague way. This was
a writing style that characterised Greenwood's approach when he
addressed a medical audience.

In his address, Greenwood emphasised the role of vital statistics
and life tables. Whilst the methods he discussed had more to do with
the life tables and actuarial work of William Farr, Greenwood was
considerably more interested in John Graunt's work on the *Natural*

and political observations upon the London Bills of Mortality.[87] Though Greenwood used Pearson's statistical methods regularly, he spent very little time talking about Pearsonian statistics to this group, which seems to have been a rather good indication of the extent to which much of the medical profession was still not predisposed to use mathematical statistics in their work.

Eight years later, Greenwood remarked that 'it came to be believed and is still believed by a majority, that epidemiology, from the scientific point of view, is a mere appendix of bacteriology, that when the means of infection and the vehicles of infection have been identified, the problems of an outbreak of herd sickness is solved'.[88] He further commented that the work of such writers as 'Farr, Brownlee and Ross are politely ignored as they are taken to be mathematical and therefore intellectually respectable, but of no practical importance'.[89]

Austin Bradford Hill and the principles of medical statistics

Greenwood's student and successor, Austin Bradford Hill (1897-1991) who had attended some of Pearson's lectures, had the greatest influence on the successful adoption of mathematical statistics in the medical community. A year after Pearson's death in 1936, the Lancet commissioned Hill to write a series of mathematical statistical articles to be published over a period of 17 weeks. Hill was indeed able to communicate statistical ideas to the medical profession with a minimal emphasis on technical details by providing a working model of medical statistics, which was based almost entirely on Pearsonian statistics. Hill 'endeavoured to make [Pearson's] statistics clear to the non-mathematically inclined worker'.[90] Shortly after C.P. Blacker began to read these articles, he wrote to Bradford Hill to congratulate him:

> on your most excellent series of articles now being published in the Lancet. I am immensely grateful to you for these. For the last ten years, I have been acutely conscious of the defects in my knowledge of these subjects. Your articles give me exactly the information that I needed in precisely the form that I wanted. I don't know how many more of these articles are destined to appear; I hope, however, that when they are completed, you will publish them as a small book. I shall purchase several copies for our Library here and will see that such a book receives a favourable review in our journal.[91]

Bradford Hill responded that

It was very kind of you to write so appreciative a letter of my articles in the Lancet. I put a great deal of work into them in the attempt to reach simplicity and to state without forbidding formulae what the statisticians is aiming at and how he goes about it. It's very gratifying to have evidence such as yours that the attempt has not been in vain. I am hoping to make a little book of the series when complete (15 or 16 in all), but that depends upon a publishers reactions. Your letter may strengthen my aim![92]

In the following year these articles were reprinted in Bradford Hill's book *The Principles of Medical Statistics* which has gone through more than nine editions. In a review of his book in the *BMJ* it was remarked that whilst Bradford Hill stressed the importance of clinical work, he also emphasised that training in statistics was also necessary for medicine. The appreciation of mathematical statistics in clinical work was, however, slow. Two reasons were cited:

The first is that the assembling of clinical or pathological data implies knowledge and experience of a special kind which have involved years of training... the other reason is that to become an expert statistician, in the technical sense, requires as much training as to become an expert clinician or pathologist... Dr Bradford Hill has provided the medical reader with the means of self-instruction. The book is short, lucid and practical.[93]

Virtually all of the statistical methods that Hill adopted were Pearson's or those of his students such as William Sealy Gosset [Student] who devised Student's t-test for independent and matched samples. This is not surprising since Hill was a student of Greenwood. The statistical methods of R.A. Fisher (1890-1960) had little to do with Hill's work. Hill did, however, choose one element of Fisher's work, a formal procedure for randomisation (which Fisher helped to popularise) and imposed it on a legacy of Pearsonian statistics and managed to make it work. Though Hill did not create any new statistical methods, his use of Pearsonian statistics for clinical trials was, nonetheless, highly innovative because this enabled him to establish the framework for the modern randomised clinical trial.[94]

Twelve years after Hill published his book, the editor of the *BMJ* commented that one of the characteristics of today's medical journals – which would certainly be not least among those which would strike the attention of the reader of half a century ago – is the increase in their statistical content and the frequent introduction of statistical methods, both elementary and highly technical.[95]

The journal looked back to the statistical methods of Galton and Pearson and remarked that the mathematical methods developed by Pearson and applied by him to biology were 'undoubtedly slow in influencing scientific thought in general and slower still in entering the medical field'. It was due to a number of Pearson's students who promulgated his statistical approach. Some of these students included John Brownlee, Major Greenwood, Raymond Pearl, Percy Stocks and George Udny Yule, all of whom used Pearsonian statistics for specifically medical problems. Clinical medicine was but little influenced, and the method of choice was still too often based upon a handful of uncontrolled cases and 'my personal experience'.[96] Yet, before this group of medical statisticians offered their services, the medical man charged with responsibility for the patient was contemptuous of the statistician's fundamental approach.

Pearson not only provided the statistical machinery for the medical profession, but more importantly a number of medical practitioners (such as Major Greenwood and John Brownlee) gained their knowledge of medical statistics by working with him in his Biometric Laboratory. Thus Pearson and his students made a difference to the way medicine used statistics by giving them a set of tools which could be adapted to suit medicine's various and constantly changing requirements.

Notes

1. Karl Pearson, ' On the influence of the sanatoriums treatment of tuberculosis', *BMJ* i (June 18, 1910), 1517.

2. P.H. Pye-Smith, 'Medicine as a science and medicine as an art' *Lancet* (1900), 310; Major Greenwood, ' Is the statistical method of any value in medical research?' *Lancet* (July 26, 1924), 158; Anon, ' Public health education' *BMJ* (November 1, 1930), 733; Anon. 'Statistics in medicine' *BMJ* (January 7, 1950), 68–9.

3. The development of Pearson's early statistical work has been examined in M. Eileen Magnello, 'Karl Pearson's Gresham Lectures: W.F.R. Weldon, speciation and the origins of Pearsonian statistics' *British Journal for the History of Science*, xxix (1996), 43–63.

4. See, for example, Lyndsay Farrall, 'The origins and growth of the English eugenics movement 1865-1926' (PhD Thesis, Indiana University, 1970); Daniel Kevles, *In the Name of Eugenics* (New York: Alfred A. Knopf, 1985); Donald Mackenzie, *Statistics in Britain 1865-1930. The Social Construction of Scientific Knowledge.* (Edinburgh: Edinburgh University Press, 1981); Bernard Norton,

'Biology and philosophy: The methodological foundation of biometry'. *Journal of the History of Biology,* vii (1975), 85–93, 92; Theodore Porter. *The Rise of Statistical Thinking* (Princeton: Princeton University Press, 1986).

5. For an assessment of a all of the methods that Pearson devised in the Biometric and the Eugenics Laboratories, in particular, see M. Eileen Magnello, ' The non-correlation of biometrics and eugenics: Rival forms of laboratory work in Karl Pearson's career at University College London', *History of Science,* xxxvii (1999), 79–106; 123–50.

6. Hawkins was at Exeter College, Oxford, was a Fellow of the Royal College of Physicians and Physician to the Westminster General Dispensary. When the Royal Statistical Society was founded in 1834, Hawkins was made a member and council member.

7. Francis Bisset Hawkins, *The Elements of Medical Statistics* (London: Longman, Rees, Orme, Brown & Green, 1829) 2.

8. *Ibid.*

9. David V. Glass, 'Two letters from the Chadwick Collection and a Correspondence between Chadwick and Farr' in David V Glass, *Numbering the People: The Eighteenth Century Population Controversy and the Development of Census and Vital Statistics in Britain.* (London: Gordon and Cremonesi, 1978; first published in 1973), 130.)

10. John Eyler, *Victorian Social Medicine. The Ideas and Methods of William Farr* (Baltimore: Johns Hopkins University Press, 1979).

11. Guy, who studied under P.C.A. Louis, received his medical degree from Cambridge in 1837 and was appointed Professor of forensic medicine at King's College London in 1838. He was honorary secretary to the Statistical Society of London from 1848-63 and vice-president from 1869-72.

12. Karl Pearson, *The Life, Letters and Labours of Francis Galton* ii (Cambridge: Cambridge University Press, 1924), 250.

13. *Ibid.*

14. Quoted from Cecil Woodham-Smith, *Florence Nightingale* (London: Constable, 1950; Reprinted 1998), 335.

15. 'Florence Nightingale, Letter to Douglas Galton (7 February 1891) in Pearson, *op. cit.* (note 12), 416.

16. *Ibid.*

17. Pearson, *op. cit.* (note 12), 418.

18. Pearson, *op. cit.* (note 12), 419–20.

19. Pearson, *op. cit.* (note 12), 416. It was only in 1988 that Oxford University renamed their Department of Biomathematics the Department of Applied Statistics.

20. For Pearson's use of matrix algebra (which he would have learned from Arthur Cayley who created matrix algebra out of his discovery of invariants during the mid-nineteenth century) see M. Eileen Magnello, 'Karl Pearson's mathematization of inheritance: from ancestral heredity to Mendelian genetics', *Annals of Science,* lv (1998), 35–94. See especially 51–5.

21. Goodness of fit tests had been used for the normal distribution by Adolphe Quetelet in 1840, Louis Adolphe Bertillon in 1863 and Galton in 1888. Pearson used his chi-square goodness of fit test with the Poisson distribution in 1927. In addition to the chi-square distribution, Gosset introduced the t-distribution in 1904 and Fisher introduced the F-distribution in 1923. These five distributions (the normal, Poisson, chi-square, *t* and *F*) became the principal theoretical distributions for modern statistical theory.

22. Galton describes the breakdown in health that he suffered during his third year at Cambridge in his *Memories of My Life* (London: Methuen and Co., 1908), 78–9.

23. Pearson's early life is examined in M. Eileen Magnello, 'Karl Pearson, elastician to biometrician: A mathematician changes contexts' in Peter Armitage and Theodore Colton (eds), *The Encyclopedia of Biostatistics,* vol. 4 (Chichester: Wiley, 1998), 3308–15.

24. On 26 May 1884, the General Board Studies decided that the short-list for the German lectureship should be limited to Karl Pearson, Mr Wolstenholme and Dr Breul. On 2 June Pearson withdrew his name and Breul was elected. I am grateful to Elisabeth Leedham, Archivist at the Cambridge University Library, for providing me with this information.

25. Karl Pearson, Letter to Oscar Browning [Written sometime between 10 October 1879 and May 1880]. Papers and correspondence of Oscar Browning, King's College Library, Cambridge.

26. The full range of Pearson's teaching at UCL is discussed in Magnello, *op. cit.* (note 5).

27. For an analysis of Pearson's early statistical work and Weldon's influence on this work, see Magnello, *op. cit.* (note 3).

28. All of Pearson's correlational methods and both of his chi-square tests are examined in Magnello, *op. cit.* (note 20), *passim.*

29. Karl Pearson, 'National life from the standpoint of science' Cavendish Lecture (Cambridge, 1912), 6.

30. Karl Pearson, Letter to Francis Galton, 1908. Papers and correspondence of Francis Galton, University College London [Hereinafter referred to as FG:UCL].

31. Pearson was quite frank with Galton in his discussions about taking

over the Eugenics Laboratory. He emphasised his reluctance in his letters of 25 October 1906, 22 December 1906 and 2 January 1908: FG:UCL. Pearson's hesitation in undertaking this laboratory is discussed in Magnello, *op. cit.* (note 5), See especially, 123–5.

32. Karl Pearson, Letter to Francis Galton, 22 December 1906. FG:UCL/293G. Reprinted in Pearson, *Life and Letters of Francis Galton,* iiia (Cambridge: Cambridge University Press, 1930), 304. The Eugenics Record Office was established in the autumn of 1904 at 50 Gower Street when Francis Galton gave the University of London £1,000 for 'the furtherance during three years of the scientific study of eugenics'. Galton supervised the office and his staff consisted of Edgar Schuster and Ethel Elderton. Pearson's role was minimal. Two years later, Schuster retired which surprised Galton who subsequently wrote to Pearson as he 'wished that the Eugenics Record Office could somehow be worked into your Biometric laboratory, but I am far too ignorant of the conditions to make a proposal'. Three weeks later Galton asked Pearson again if he could be 'persuaded to take control of the Eugenics office as a branch of the Biometric Laboratory'.

33. Though Pearson's statistical work has been inextricably linked to Galton and to the work undertaken in the Eugenics Laboratory, Pearson, in fact, made very little use of his biometric methods in this Laboratory. Indeed Pearson recognised the limitations of his biometric methods for problems of eugenics. He developed instead a completely separate methodology for problems relating to eugenics. See Magnello, *op. cit.* (note 5).

34. Karl Pearson, 'Report on certain enteric fever inoculation statistics', *BMJ* (5 November 1904), 1243–6.

35. Karl Pearson, 'Mathematical contributions to the theory of evolution. VII. On the correlation of 119characters not quantitatively measurable' *Philosophical Transactions of the Royal Society,* ser. A, cxcv (1900), 79–250, 142.

36. William Fleetwood Sheppard, 'On the application to the theory of error to cases of normal distribution and normal correlation', *Philosophical Transactions of the Royal Society,* ser. A, cxcii (1898), 167, Table VI.

37. The values of the phi coefficient range from -1 to +1. Pearson's statistical methods of correlation and association are examined more fully in Magnello, *op. cit.* (note 20), 62–6. Also see Magnello *op. cit.* (note 5) Table 4, 96.

38. Karl Pearson, 'Report on certain enteric fever inoculation statistics', *BMJ* (5 November 1904) 1243–46, 1245.

39. For the *BMJ's* support of Pearson, see Leader, 'Antityphoid
    inoculation' *BMJ* (5 November 1904), 1259-61, 1260. Rosser
    Matthews examines this debate in his *Quantification and the Quest
    for Medical Certainty* (Princeton: Princeton University Press, 1995).
    See Chapter 5. For an account of Wright's work on vaccine therapy
    see Michael Worboys, 'Vaccine therapy and laboratory medicine in
    Edwardian Britain' in John Pickstone (ed.), *Medical Innovations in
    Historical Perspective* (Manchester: Manchester University Press,
    1992), 84–103.
40. See especially Richard Peto, M.C. Pike, Peter Armitage, N.E.
    Breslow, D.R. Cox, S.V. Howard, N Mantel, K. McPherson, J. Peto
    and P.G. Smith 'Design and analysis of randomized clinical trials
    requiring prolonged observations of each patient I. Introduction and
    Design', *British Journal of Cancer*, xxxiv (1976), 585–612. 'Part II.
    Analysis and Examples' xxxv (1977), 2–37.
41. Michael Worboys, 'The sanatorium treatment for consumption in
    Britain, 1890-1914' in John Pickstone, *op. cit.* (note 39), 47–71, 49.
42. Karl Pearson, 'A first study of the statistics of pulmonary
    tuberculosis', *Drapers' Company Research Memoirs. Studies in National
    Deterioration,* II (1907) 26. Also see G. Norman Meachen, *A Short
    History of Tuberculosis,* (London, 1936) 56.
43. Karl Pearson, 'The inheritance of insanity' *BMJ,* (May 27, 1905),
    1175–6.
44. *Ibid.*, 1176.
45. Karl Pearson, 'On the influence of the sanatoriums treatment of
    tuberculosis', *BMJ* 1 (June 18, 1910), 1517.
46. *Ibid.*
47. Karl Pearson, 'Heredity and environment' *BMJ,* (July 9, 1910), 117.
48. Karl Pearson, Letter to Major Greenwood, (14 July 1910)
    KP:UCL/915.
49. James Barr, Letter to Karl Pearson (30 May 1914) KP:UCL/630/5.
50. Wm. S Paget-Tomlinson ' Sanatorium treatment of tuberculosis'
    BMJ (23 July 1910), 225–6 and John Guy, Letter to the Editor,
    BMJ (23 July 1910), 227.
51. Paget-Tomlinson, *op. cit.* (note 50), 225. Also see Worboys, *op. cit.*
    (note 41).
52. Paget-Tomlinson, *op. cit.* (note 50). 226.
53. John Guy, Letter to the Editor, *BMJ* (23 July 1910) 227.
54. Karl Pearson , 'Sanatorium treatment of tuberculosis' *BMJ,* (August
    6, 1910) 349.
55. *Ibid,* 349.
56. Karl Pearson, Sanatorium treatment of consumption' *BMJ* (August

27, 1910) 570–1.

57. *Ibid.*, 570

58. *Ibid.*, 571.

59. Karl Pearson, 'Sanatorium treatment of tuberculosis' *BMJ* (September 24, 1910), 906.

60. Pearson, *op. cit.* (note 56), 906.

61. Philip Henry Pye-Smith, 'Medicine as science, and medicine as art', *Lancet* (August 4, 1900), 309–12: 310.

62. Anon., 'Recent Advances in statistical methods' *BMJ* (July 13, 1907), 95–8.

63. *Ibid.*, 98.

64. James MacDonald Troup and G. Darell Maynard, ' Modern Statistical Methods' *Lancet*, (May 14, 1910), 1336–43.

65. *Ibid.*, 1343.

66. Anon., 'Modern statistical methods" *BMJ* (August 13, 1910), 393.

67. *Ibid.*

68. Anon., 'Mathematics and medicine', *BMJ* (August 26, 1911), 449.

69. For the *BMJ's* view on Ross, see *ibid.*

70. Anon., *op. cit.* (note 68), 449.

71. For an analysis of Ross's contributions to epidemiology see David J Bradley, 'The intellectual legacies of Ronald Ross' *Indian journal of malariology*, cccxliv (1997), 73–5.

72. Anon., *op. cit.* (note 68)

73. Ronald Ross, Letter to Karl Pearson (30 June 1905). Papers and correspondence of Karl Pearson, University College London/126 [Hereinafter referred to as KP:UCL]. Ross also expressed his concern in a letter to the editor on 'The possibility of reducing mosquitoes', *Nature*, (June 15, 1905), 151.

74. See Karl Pearson, 'The problem of the random walk' *Nature*, lxxii (1905), 294 and 342.

75. Ronald Ross, Letter to Karl Pearson (24 July 1905) KP:UCL/126.

76. Anon, 'Science notes' *BMJ* (November 4, 1911) 1210. Also see Karl Pearson and John Blakeman, 'Mathematical contribution to the theory of evolution. XV. A mathematical theory of random migration', *Drapers' Company Research Memoirs. Biometric Series. III* (1906), 54–105.

77. The resistance met by the Mendelians is discussed by Magnello, *op. cit.* (note 20).

78. Major Greenwood, Letter to Karl Pearson (18 March 1902), KP:UCL/707.

79. Karl Pearson, Letter to Major Greenwood (22 September 1904), KP:UCL/915.

80. Karl Pearson, Letter to Major Greenwood (14 July 1910), KP:UCL/915.
81. Major Greenwood, Letter to Karl Pearson (18 July 1910), KP:UCL/395.
82. *Ibid.*
83. [Major Greenwood and Karl Pearson] ' Memorandum on the need for statistical training in the medical curriculum' [1922], KP:UCL/707.
84. *Ibid.*
85. Karl Pearson, 'Report to the Court of the Worshipful Company of Drapers for the years 1922, 1923 and 1924'. KP:UCL/283.
86. Major Greenwood, ' Is the statistical method of any value in medical research?' *Lancet* (July 26, 1924), 153–8.
87. *Ibid.* See especially 154–6. Also see Captain John Graunt, 'The epistle dedicatory of *Natural and Political Observations upon the Bills of Mortality* [1662] in Charles Henry Hull, *Economic Writings of Sir William Petty with the Natural and Political Observations upon the Bills of Mortality (more probably by John Graunt)* vol. II (Cambridge: Cambridge University Press, 1899).
88. Major Greenwood, *Epidemiology: Historical and experimental* (Baltimore: Johns Hopkins University Press, 1932), 18–9
89. *Ibid.*, 19.
90. Austin Bradford Hill, 'I. The aim of the statistical method' *Lancet* (2 January 1937), 47.
91. C.P. Blacker, Letter to Austin Bradford Hill (23 February 1937), Archive of Eugenics Society, Wellcome Library [SA/EUG/G/C.152].
92. A. Bradford Hill to C.P. Blacker (24 February 1937) Archive of Eugenics Society, Wellcome Library [SA/EUG/G/C.152].
93. Anon. 'Medical Statistics', *BMJ*, (September 18, 1937) 583.
94. For a comprehensive analysis of the development of the clinical trial see Desirée Cox-Maksimov, 'The making of the clinical trial in Britain, 1910-1945: Expertise, the State and the Public' (PhD Thesis, Cambridge, 1997). The work of Peter Armitage and Richard Peto in the 1970s helped to make Fisherian statistics more accessible for medical research. See especially Richard Peto, M.C. Pike, Peter Armitage, N.E. Breslow, D.R. Cox, S.V. Howard, N Mantel, K. McPherson, J. Peto and P.G. Smith 'Design and analysis of randomized clinical trials requiring prolonged observations of each patient. Part I. Introduction and design' *British Journal of Cancer,* xxxiv (1976), 585–612. 'Part II. Analysis and examples' xxxv (1977), 2–37.
95. Anon., 'Statistics in medicine' *BMJ*, (January 7, 1950), 68–9.
96. *Ibid.*

6

Almroth Wright, Vaccine Therapy
and British Biometrics:

Disciplinary Expertise versus Statistical Objectivity[1]

J. Rosser Matthews

With the advent of bacteriology in the late-nineteenth century, the question of whether medicine was a laboratory-based science or a clinical art was brought to the forefront of medical debate; physicians would now face a tension in social and professional roles of how to divide their time between the bedside and the laboratory bench. Even though the introduction of laboratory techniques created a sense of professional ambivalence (that has persisted to this day), there was actually much uniting the clinician and bacteriologist when their approach to medical judgment is viewed through the filter of another point of view – that of the biometrician. By adopting a thoroughgoing quantitative approach, the biometrician aimed at making medical judgment fully explicit whereas the bacteriologist (like the clinician) emphasised the role of acquired disciplinary expertise on the part of the medical researcher. In this paper, I will illustrate this divergence in the point of view as evidenced by the debate over the value of vaccine therapy between the bacteriologist Sir Almroth Wright (1861–1947) and Karl Pearson's biometrical school in the first decades of the twentieth century, as well as speculate on how this debate within medicine reflects differing views about the nature of scientific reasoning and its role in twentieth century society and culture.

Wright's early training clearly illustrates the growing prestige of laboratory methods for the aspiring bacteriologist. After graduating from Trinity College Dublin in 1883, he was awarded a travelling fellowship of £100 to visit the University of Leipzig where he studied under such pioneers as Julius Cohnheim, Carl Weigert, and Carl Ludwig. Upon his return to the British Isles, he held various positions including working as a demonstrator in Michael Foster's physiological laboratory at Cambridge before receiving a Grocers' Company scholarship in 1888 to return to Germany for further study. From 1889 to 1891, he served as a demonstrator in physiology at Sydney, Australia before returning to England permanently. In 1892, he was appointed professor of pathology at the Royal Army Medical College, Netley where he developed an immunisation serum against typhoid fever that proved to be the subject of much controversy between Wright, the medical profession, and Karl Pearson (1857–1936).[2]

In 1902, Wright was appointed pathologist at St. Mary's Hospital, Paddington where he subsequently founded an inoculation department to provide an institutional base for his researches into vaccine therapy. The principal means that Wright developed for testing the efficacy of these inoculation procedures was what he termed the 'opsonic index'. With his associate Stewart Douglas, Wright discovered that there was a substance in blood serum (opsonin) that prepared bacteria to be ingested by the leucocytes (white blood corpuscles). In a normal person the amount of opsonin remained constant, but in persons attacked by a bacterial substance, there soon resulted either an increase or a decrease of the opsonin in the blood serum. By measuring a patient's opsonic index at regular intervals, Wright hoped to demonstrate the efficacy of various vaccines, i.e., if vaccination brought an individual's opsonic index into the normal range, the procedure had been successful at inducing immunity.

The experimental procedure for measuring the opsonic index proved to be complex: quantities of the patient's serum, a suspension of microbes, and a suspension of normal leucocytes were mixed together and kept at body temperature for half an hour. Then a preparation of the mixture was made on a glass slide, stained with an appropriate dye, examined under a microscope, and the number of microbes seen in each leucocyte counted. From 25 to 100 leucocytes were examined, the number of microbes in each leucocyte was noted, and the average number of microbes per leucocyte was then computed. A similar procedure was then carried out on a normal person as a control. The ratio of these two average values constituted the opsonic index, i.e., if there were no difference between the two individuals, then the opsonic index would be close to unity. In general, Wright maintained that if the ratio went below 0.8 or above 1.2, then infection with that microbe was usually found. By these means, Wright had hoped to detect infections before the individual displayed any clinical manifestations of disease.[3]

Since Wright's procedure involved comparing two average values (what the statistically-trained person would call a mean), his method was seized upon by Karl Pearson and his biometrical followers at

University College London who were attempting to reconstitute statistics as an applied mathematical discipline; the statistical critique of the opsonic index helped to launch the career of one of Pearson's medical students – Major Greenwood (1880–1949). In a 1909 presentation before the pathological section of the Royal Society of Medicine, Greenwood outlined what he saw as the principal flaw of Wright's method: the skewness of the distribution produced when one plotted a frequency diagram of the number of microbes found in each leucocyte. As a result of this asymmetry, Greenwood observed that the mode, or most frequently occurring value, would be a better constant than the mean. In addition to these specifically mathematical criticisms, Greenwood's analysis was also important for outlining what would become a key point of contention between Wright and the biometricians – the distinction between errors of technique that would cause incorrect facts to be recorded and mathematical error that derived from the fact that conclusions were based on a sample rather than the population as a whole. For Greenwood, errors of technique were the province of the medical researcher and errors of random sampling were the province of the statistician.[4]

Other associates of Pearson not only echoed Greenwood's views but also emphasised how statistical methods made it no longer necessary for medical researchers to appeal to the amorphous concept of personal 'experience' when discussing therapeutic efficacy. As W. F. Harvey and Anderson McKendrick observed in an article in *Biometrika*:

> The improvement in the condition of the patient expressed in terms of feeling-of-well-being, the check in the spread of disease processes, the extension in the duration of life produced by particular methods of treatment have scarcely at all been taken into account because they are not available in a form suitable for statistical treatment. These data may be grouped under the commonly used term, experience. But experience is largely a personal matter and can only carry limited weight in argument or at most appeal to the comparatively few....

> ...[I]f over a wide range of diseases ... there would seem to be accumulating evidence in favour of the arrival of a new era of treatment we may reasonable anticipate that these hopes will ultimately prove, if properly recorded, to be based on statistically significant foundations. But we must discard the *fetish of experience* [my emphasis], and set to work at the expense of some labour to

127

record the essence of that experience so that all the world may judge of its real value. The work requires co-operation, and the realisation of this fact may speed the advance of exact measurement in the domain of medicine.[5]

As an individual trained in laboratory methods, Wright had no interest in abandoning the 'fetish of experience' in medical judgment. Rather, his scientific writings continually emphasised experimentation as the key to intellectual insight. As Wright noted in his 1906 textbook *The Principles of Microscopy*: 'If . . . the reader sees ground of complaint in the fact that he is required at every moment to put down the book and undertake an experiment, I would submit that no proposition is adequately apprehended until it has been invested in the apposite mental image.' Mathematics, by contrast, was downplayed: 'the use of mathematical signs as a substitute for speech can be defended only in the case of the inarticulate classes of the learned.'[6] Despite such programmatic assertions, Wright did not find mathematics totally useless (the opsonic index was, after all, a mathematical construct); however, his preference for experimental intervention rather than mathematical manipulation was beyond doubt.

For this reason, Wright placed much greater emphasis on minimising errors of technique (what he called 'functional errors') than on errors that derived from the problem of random sampling (what he called 'mathematical errors'). As he observed in a speech on vaccine therapy before the Royal Society of Medicine in May of 1910:

> I have satisfied myself, and all my fellow-workers have satisfied themselves, and I am glad to say a very large and increasing number of bacteriological workers all over the world have satisfied themselves, that when the 'functional error' has been reduced, as it can be by practice and patience, to small dimensions and when, in connexion with tubercle, the customary counts of 100 or more leucocytes are made, the 'mathematical limit of error' of the opsonic index is such as need not seriously be taken into account.[7]

In a letter to Greenwood later in the year, Wright emphasised further how even his terminology of 'functional' error underlined the central importance of personal expertise: 'I have venture[d] to coin the term 'functional error' because 'personal equation' suggests that there is an unvarying functional error for each operator which he cannot improve upon.' However, Wright declared that his primary focus on functional error did not mean that he denied the need for statistical results; he told Greenwood that he 'had no polemical end' and that his writings were intended 'merely as a preliminary enquiry into the logical basis of our method. Witness what I have said about the demand that we should gain statistical results for our treatment when we cannot agree as to what the verdict is to be in the individual case.'[8]

Despite Wright's concessions regarding the need for statistical results, his belief that individual expertise could still overrule insights drawn from multiple observations was anathema to Karl Pearson on both political and scientific grounds. As a socialist by political persuasion, Pearson believed that the individual had to subordinate his or her desires to the larger social good; as he observed in his popular treatise *The Grammar of Science*, 'the tribal conscience ought for the sake of social welfare to be stronger than private interest.' Similarly, Pearson believed that the individual insights of the scientist were less important than the patterns that emerged from multiple statistical observations; for Pearson, science consisted in the 'classification of facts and the formation of absolute judgments independent of the idiosyncrasies of the individual mind.'[9] Several notable consequences followed from Pearson's views. Specifically, science was seen as a method of classification that could be applied with equal validity to all types of aggregative phenomena – both natural and social. Also, to ensure that an inference was truly scientific (in the sense of untainted by individual beliefs), Pearson required that it be an inference 'which could be drawn by every logically trained normal mind, if it were in possession of the conceptions upon which the inference has been based'.[10] Thus, Pearson's scientific and political philosophies proved to opposite sides of the same coin; both held up the ideal of minimising the importance of individual judgment. As Theodore M. Porter has claimed, this core political vision of the 'disappearing subject' or the *unrettbar Ich* underlay Pearson's entire philosophy and scientific career.[11]

As a matter of philosophical conviction, therefore, Pearson felt obliged to respond to Wright's assertion that the 'mathematical' error from random sampling 'need not seriously be taken into account' when the 'functional' error of the individual experimenter had been reduced to a minimum. In an article in *Biometrika*, Pearson acknowledged that Wright had 'very properly' pointed out that variation in the opsonic index depended on 'the functional error of the individual observer' and the 'error of method' (i.e., mathematical error); however, he took exception to Wright's claims that

The 'functional error' is an error which attaches only to methods which involve a certain amount of skilful function. It attaches to the *operator* [italics in original]. It may in the case of one and the same operator vary from hour to hour with his physiological efficiency. Its value can be diminished by practice and attention. It cannot be evaluated by a mathematician. It can be pretty accurately gauged by the operator himself.[12]

Such declarations of individual expertise ran completely counter to Pearson's vision of the nature of the scientific enterprise. As Pearson observed:

[I]t is difficult to see wherein the functional error of the vaccine therapy observer differs from that of the astronomical observer. His personal equation also varies from hour to hour with his physiological efficiency and it has a different value for every operator. What sort of reply would Gauss and Bessel have given to the astronomer who said that his functional error could not 'be evaluated by a mathematician', but could be 'pretty accurately gauged' by himself? Have we not here an instance of how disastrous is the specialisation of modern science, which so completely prevents a distinguished specialist from knowing the history of branches of science outside his own little field?... The insistence of Sir Almroth Wright on the distinction between variations due to random samples and variations due to observational skill is perfectly legitimate and of vital importance, but his argument that the one and not the other is capable of exact treatment shows ... [the] limitation of his knowledge of statistical methods.[13]

In a statement that would soon become a key bone of contention between himself and Wright, Pearson declared that 'the day of authority in any branch of science has gone by, and we ask legitimately and instinctively for the data from which this satisfaction was extracted'.[14]

Pearson then proceeded to analyse three different data sets involving opsonic index measurements. The data had been collected by Alexander Fleming who worked in Wright's laboratory (and later became famous as the discoverer of penicillin), Major Greenwood and J. D. C. White who worked in Pearson's biometrical laboratory, and T. S. P. Strangeways. In the first two instances, Pearson worked with data sets in which a total of 1,000 bacilli had been observed in the leucocytes so that he could plot the resulting frequency distributions with bacilli per leucocyte on the horizontal axis and the frequency with which each ratio of bacilli per leucocyte occurred on the vertical axis. In the case of Fleming's data, the mean number of bacilli per leucocyte was 3.72, the mode was 2.67, and the standard deviation was 2.40; for Greenwood and White's data, the mean was 3.61, the mode was 1.94, and the standard deviation was 2.59. Since Strangeways had counted 2000 single cells as well as 3000 clumped cells, Pearson was able to generate 40 samples of 50 cells each (for the single cells) and 60 samples of 50 (for the clumped cells). Strangeways's results could then be compared directly with Greenwood's and White's 400 samples of 50 (i.e., for a total of 20,000 cells). Strangeways's data generated a mean opsonic indices of 1.0202 (single cells) and 1.0221 (clumped cells) whereas Greenwood's and White's data generated a mean opsonic index of 1.0205; the corresponding mode values were 0.9852, 0.9734, and 0.9611; the corresponding standard deviations were 0.2083, 0.2181, and 0.2072 respectively. On the basis of the closeness in value of the relevant constants for all investigators, Pearson concluded:

> there is no significant difference in the variation of these three series; no one of them can be described as having 'enormous working errors' compared with another; they show, for arguments about the range of variation of the opsonic index, practically equivalent results . . . The only conclusion that anyone examining . . . the above analytical constants of the curves, can reach, is that: If the countings are done by different microscopists, not members of Sir Almroth Wright's Laboratory, the variation in the opsonic index of an individual reckoned against himself shows the same magnitude of range, and this whether the slide was prepared or not in Sir Almroth's Laboratory.[15]

In view of the fact that there was no appreciable difference in the variation of the opsonic index regardless of who collected or analysed the data, Pearson concluded (as an 'unprejudiced outsider') that 'a claim to special monopoly of technique in placing the film on the slide or in preparing it in any way needs further justification.'[16] In a clear statement of his view that the essence of science lay in appeals to statistical methods, Pearson declared that:

> it is scarcely scientific – without publishing evidence of any kind – to appeal vaguely to the 'satisfaction' of 'a large and increasing number of bacteriological workers all over the world.' Statistics on the table, please! I may be quite in error, but at any rate the evidence on which my conclusions are based is here provided for criticism and correction.[17]

Wright responded to the arguments of the biometricians in several publications that appeared in 1912. In an appendix to his *Handbook of the Technique of the Teat and Capillary Glass Tube*, Wright openly acknowledged the statistician's point that there existed a 'factor of chance' since averages were computed from samples which contained opsonic indices that varied over a range of values. However, he still took exception to the statistician being the sole arbiter of what constituted a 'significant' result, that is, a result in which the difference between two groups of figures was 'due to causes other than the operation of chance'.[18]

Wright observed:

> They [the statisticians] suggest that there is to be found somewhere a sharp dividing line between what is probable and what is improbable, and between what is worth taking into consideration and what is not worth taking into consideration; and they suggest to the ordinary reader that the mathematical statistician who uses the terms has scientific resources at his disposal which justify him in affirming with respect to differences which fall within certain limits that they are due to the operation of chance, and in dictating that such differences – even though they may be constantly recurring in significant connexions – should be simply wiped off the record and discarded.

> It cannot be too clearly understood that the mathematical statistician has no such secret wells of wisdom to draw from, and that his science does not justify his going one step beyond the purely numerical statement that – as computed by him from the data he has selected as suitable for his purposes – the probabilities in favour of a particular difference being or not being due to the operation of chance are such and such.

> There need, therefore, be no hesitation in saying that when the mathematical statistician makes free with the terms *significant* and *non-significant*, he is simply taking upon himself a function to which he can lay no claim in his capacity of a mathematician.

> It is his proper function to compute the probabilities, it belongs to the practical man of affairs – in connexion with the opsonic index, to the practical doctor – to decide whether a particular degree of probability may, for the purposes of practical life, be allowed to rank as a certainty.[19]

Clearly, Wright believed that his 'practical' insights as a physician and experimenter could override the 'theoretical' concerns of the statistician.

By the time his textbook had appeared, Wright had turned his attention to the question of pneumococcal vaccine after being appointed as a paid consultant to the Rand Mines in South Africa. With the discovery of gold and diamonds in South Africa in the last decades of the nineteenth century, large numbers of black mine workers had been 'recruited' to work the mines often from distant regions of Africa. As a result of the harsh working conditions and the arduous transport to the mines, many contracted pneumonia as well as sinusitis, meningitis and pericarditis. When Wright arrived in South Africa, he attempted to use the miners as a test case to prove the efficacy of vaccine therapy; he immunised nearly 50,000 natives in 1911–12 by injecting them with randomly obtained, killed pneumococci.[20]

Wright published the preliminary results of his findings in two articles that appeared in the *Lancet* at the end of 1912; these articles not only outlined Wright's method of research, they also provided another opportunity for Wright to elaborate philosophically on why he rejected the biometricians' arguments. Initially, Wright discussed the use of a new experimental drug (aethylhydrocupreinhydrochlorate) for pneumococcal infections. After testing the drug on mice, Wright reported on its effects on three natives by measuring changes in their opsonic indices at a regular interval (3 hrs.) after receiving the drug. In general, Wright concluded that 'the *opsonic power* of the serum is not appreciably affected by the exhibition of the drug'.[21] Then Wright moved from his particular empirical conclusions to the more general question of how one establishes therapeutic efficacy. He maintained that there was either the method of 'crucial experiment' (an experiment which always yields the same conclusion and, therefore, may be regarded as a 'universal truth') or the method of 'cumulative experiment' wherein 'we have to experiment in conditions which cannot be sufficiently simplified to allow of the institution of a crucial experiment.' Wright then asserted that cumulative experiments could be evaluated either by means of the 'experiential method' (i.e., the experimenter takes into account 'the whole complex of impressions which been left upon the mind by experience') or the 'statistical method' (the experimenter records the percentage of cases in which a particular result has been achieved).[22]

By introducing these methodological distinctions in the order that he did, Wright clearly implied a procedural hierarchy with 'crucial experiments' as the most desirable method and 'statistical methods' as the least. In further elaborating on the distinction between experiential and statistical methods, Wright observed:

In the case of an *experiential evaluation,* the position is as follows: We have no real guarantee for the inclusion of every case in the record. On the other hand, we can feel confident that no significant factor has been excluded from consideration, and that, so far as possible, credit has been given for every such factor. Thus, for example, we may, where the recovery of the patient counts as a success, feel sure that proportionately more credit will have been allowed to a rapid and triumphant recovery; and proportionately less to a slow and incomplete recovery.

In a case of a *statistical evaluation,* the position is almost the reverse. We have here a very strong presumption – for the keeping of a statistical table affords such a presumption – that the result of every case has come upon the record. On the other hand, we know that no significant element except that which serves as the basis of classification has been brought into the account. And, in the case where the presence or absence of a critical feature provides the basis of classification, we know that the evaluation is inaccurate in the respect that there has been assigned to each case, according as it fell above or below an arbitrary line, either the absolute maximum of marks, or no marks at all.[23]

Once again, Wright's reasons for favouring experiential over statistical evaluation centred on the issue of personal expertise. Since experiential evaluation permitted one to take all factors into consideration (including clinical uncertainties), the researcher could arrive at more accurate conclusions. Statistical evaluation, by contrast, could not account for such uncertainties since the method required that each case be definitively assigned to one category or another. As Wright observed in the case of statistics of pneumonia, 'We are ... compelled to accept it that every man who is set down as having died of pneumonia really died of it. And, of course, we are compelled to accept it that there were not among the cases which came under observation any cases where the diagnosis was doubtful.'[24] Thus, by failing to recognise such diagnostic uncertainties (which the experienced clinician would have perceived intuitively), the method of statistical evaluation presented only the false appearance of objectivity, a fact which might lead to incorrect conclusions.

From these general observations on the relative merits of experiential and statistical evaluation, Wright moved to the specific issue of Pearson's assertion that the scientific method was, at its core, statistical. In discussing this issue, Wright was self-consciously aware of the normative and political underpinnings that informed Pearson's point of view; he framed the issue by posing the question 'Do considerations of intellectual morality prescribe that the statistical method should everywhere be brought into application?' Wright then outlined the essential features of Pearson's philosophy thus:

> the statistical method is believed to provide effective safeguards against moral shortcomings on the part of the observer and the evaluator – shortcomings such as a departure from impartiality; a holding back of facts which ought to be disclosed; and a laying claim to unwarranted authority. The statistical method does, in point of fact, offer against these certain safeguards ...

> In considerations of these facts the statistical method has come to stand for certain moral ideas. It stands for the ideal of clearing one's mind of bias; for the ideal of making a full disclosure of the facts, and submitting all one's data to the court of appeal of one's fellow-workers; and for the ideal of disclaiming all authority except that derived from the observations one has actually put on record.[25]

Even though Wright clearly regarded the statistical method as possessing some merit, he took exception to Pearson's claim that the statistical approach should become the *sine qua non* in deciding all scientific issues. In response to Pearson's assertion that 'The day of authority in any branch of science has gone by', Wright observed:

> The scientific observer is here told in almost so many words that he must never presume to enunciate an experiential conclusion in any authoritative tone; that he must never, even in the case where he happens to be an expert claim to be listened to except on the ground that he has been the vehicle through which a certain number of data have been put on record; and that, so long as he employs the experiential method, it is not allowable for him to maintain his opinion against even a quite non-authoritative worker who employs the statistical method.[26]

Wright found such a denial of individual expertise abhorrent largely because it did fundamental violence to his conception of medicine as a profession. He characterised Pearson's view as 'socialistic egalitarianism in science' and affirmed that 'this doctrine cannot find application in medicine; for here in many cases truth can be arrived at only by *exceptional skill* [my emphasis] and a very delicate calculation of probabilities'. In addition, Wright maintained that a uniform statistical methodology would fundamentally alter the character of medicine; the statistically-trained would no longer have to be mindful of the Hippocratic admonition: *Experientia fallax, judicium difficile.* Finally, Wright observed that, when one reflected on the 'armchair statistician' who 'ruled out all authority in science saving only that of his craft', it quickly became apparent

> that the wheel has come full circle, and that the programme of socialistic egalitarianism – the programme of abolishing in every branch of science the despotism of the expert – has ended in the setting up the statistician as dictator wherever in any part of the field of knowledge the method of cumulative experiment comes into application.

> When it is made a matter of reproach against the experiential method that it encourages scientific workers who have served a full apprenticeship to arrogate to themselves unwarranted authority in their special department of observation or experiment; let it be borne in mind that the statistical method encourages the comparatively inexperienced observer to put forward his evaluations as final; and that it invites the man who only collects and digests other men's observations to assume the role of a universal arbiter and final referee.[27]

Wright had realised (correctly) that to subject his medical judgment to the tribunal of statistical criticism constituted an abdication of his disciplinary authority as a physician.

As one would expect, Pearson did not accept Wright's assertions and advised his former student Major Greenwood to respond to Wright's claims publicly in view of the fact Wright's views had now become known to the wider medical community. As Pearson observed in a letter to Greenwood:

> I had seen Wright in the Lancet. My feeling on reading his 'Report' originally was precisely that I had when I read his reply to me on Enteric Inoculation – i.e., that he was fighting for something more substantial than truth. He has gone out to S. Africa, not to study as a statistician would the facts of pneumonia among the miners, and he has so I understand failed because he has not correlated cause & effect, each phase of environment with the mortality. He has come back irritated & wished to attach the method he has neglected.[28]

Pearson further advised Greenwood that 'It might be well to point out that the very idea of the opsonic index was to extend the quantitative appreciation of symptoms and to obtain comparisons more definite than mere 'authoritative' opinion.'[29]

Greenwood was well positioned professionally to take on Wright. After receiving his license to practice medicine and studying under Pearson during the academic year 1904/5, Greenwood had been awarded a research scholarship by the British Medical Association and became the demonstrator in Leonard Hill's physiological laboratory in the London Hospital Medical School working on caisson disease.[30] In 1909, the director of the Lister Institute of Preventive Medicine, Charles James Martin, had established a full-time position for him as head of a newly-created statistical department; this was the first post in Great Britain that was expressly created to deal with medical subjects biometrically. Greenwood had assumed this post on 1 January 1910 and had resigned his position of demonstrator of physiology; however, he retained his position as head of the London Hospital Statistical Department so that he would have the requisite access to statistical records.[31] Thus, Greenwood possessed both statistical and laboratory training thereby making him uniquely qualified to respond to Wright's assertions on the relative merits of each approach. As he wrote to Pearson shortly before assuming his statistical post: 'I don't regret my physiological work, it has enabled me to meet the enemy who talks about arm-chair statisticians on his own ground.'[32]

In his response to Wright in the *Lancet*, Greenwood addressed (with varying degrees of intellectual sophistication) Wright's main arguments – the appropriation of the term *significant* by the statistician, the superiority of the 'experiential' method over the 'statistical' one, the belief in 'crucial experiments' to decide uncertain scientific issues, and the role of individual expertise in making scientific judgments. On the issue of the use of the term *significant*, Greenwood was dismissive. He maintained that the statistician had never claimed that the standard was absolute and cited one of his own previous papers in which he had declared that 'each must judge for himself what limit of probability to take as a standard, but it is well to remember that such standard is, in some measure, arbitrary'. In addition, Greenwood held that Wright's accusations consisted of more or less serious misrepresentations of what the statisticians really did.

> This seems to be due to a very superficial examination of the work stigmatised, and suggests that Sir Almroth Wright has either read the papers in questions carelessly or is unable to comprehend them. The adoption of either alternative goes far to discredit the claim he, in effect, makes to sit in judgment upon the applicability of statistical

methods to medical problems.[33]

Ultimately, the question of 'significance' did not prove to be an issue on which Wright and Greenwood engaged in 'significant' intellectual debate; their exchange basically consisted of mutual *ad hominem* attacks.

On the question of the relative merits of the 'experiential' and the 'statistical' method, Greenwood effectively turned Wright on his head. Whereas Wright had praised the experiential method over the statistical for the former's attention to all relevant factors rather than just what could be counted, Greenwood emphasised the value of a statistical approach for overcoming the inadequacy of sense perception. He observed:

> It is the experience of everyday life that the same external stimulus does not always call up the same sensation, and that different stimuli may elicit an identical response. What alchemy of medical experience can free the expert in that science from the ordinary weakness? Surely it is the universal recognition of this which makes a disclosure of the evidence a first principle in non-medical scientific work? We all admit that in any complex of sense impressions there may be some which it is difficult or impossible to place on the record, but the fact that we have not within ourselves any constant standard of measuring these fleeting impressions deprives them of logical validity.[34]

Like his mentor Karl Pearson, Greenwood repudiated as unscientific any 'fleeting impressions' based on only individual judgment.

On the question of existence of a 'crucial experiment', Greenwood provided a more substantive response. By drawing on his own experiences as a 'sometime demonstrator in physiology', Greenwood described a common experiment in which three test tubes were prepared: the first contained fibrin, glycerin extract of pig's stomach, and water; the second substituted 0.2 percent solution of hydrochloric acid for the water; and the third was the same as the second except for the omission of the gastric extract. The three tubes were incubated at body temperature for half an hour at which time the student observed that fibrin had partly disappeared from the second tube and was unchanged in the first and third tubes thereby implying that the presence of acid was the decisive factor. Although the demonstrator always obtained the same result when this experiment was performed, Greenwood concluded that the experiment is 'strictly more of the nature of a demonstration than a proof'. In order to establish a proof of the experimental result, Greenwood emphasised that the experiment had to be repeated on multiple occasions:

> Let us place ourselves in the position of the physiologist who, moved, let us say, by some speculation, first performed the experiment, would he have been justified in straightway proclaiming that he had proved the point? Suppose some serious therapeutic issue turned on an answer to the question, Is gastric proteolysis possible in the absence of mineral acid? would he be justified in taking action upon the strength of a single crucial experiment (assuming even that all his materials were chemically pure)? The answer is, of course, No, and Sir Almroth Wright recognises this ...
>
> ...Were Sir Almroth Wright better acquainted with the history of mathematical statistics, he would know that a problem closely akin to this one is a classic of the science.[35]

Finally, on the question of the role of 'authoritative' opinion in science, Greenwood responded by coining a distinction between the grounds of *action* and the grounds of *proof*.[36] In describing the grounds of action, he used the example of calling in a medical expert when one's child becomes sick. If the medical expert 'X' was highly recommended by one's personal physician as well as others, then one was entitled as a ground of action to accept the recommendation of 'X' at face value: 'The conclusion emerges that I ought to follow X's advice – that is to say, the competence of X, the only matter respecting which I have evidence, is sufficiently established to form a ground of action for me.'[37] On the practical matter of what should be done in a specific case, Greenwood had no problem with utilising professional expertise; however, on the theoretical question of 'the cogency of the reasons which justified X's action in that case', Greenwood did not feel that basing judgments merely on the consensus of expert opinion was warranted in any way. As he observed, neither expert nor non-expert would then possess any ground of proof that X's assertions were justified:

> Suppose that X obstinately confines himself to the argument that his experience and that of fellow experts prove that his opinion would be correct in the vast majority of such cases, then the non-medical scientific man is permanently deprived of any ground of *proof*. It is likely, is indeed of everyday occurrence that he will now fall into the error, mentioned by Sir Almroth Wright, of comparing things not *in pari materia*. He will note the utterances of X with respect to other

matters, say votes for women, and if he finds that X talks nonsense or draws illogical inferences with respect to that question, the *materia* of which is non-medical, may hastily conclude that X's surgical inferences are not better founded. But not only is the non-expert destitute of valid grounds of proof; the expert is in hardly better case. He cannot be sure that he attaches the same meaning to the words 'great majority of cases', 'consensus of opinion', 'teaching of experience', as another expert. He is unable to fulfil the requirement of a valid scientific inference – viz. That it is such as 'could be drawn by every logically trained normal mind if it were in possession of the conceptions upon which the inference has been based.'[38]

In elaborating on the grounds of proof, Greenwood provided one of the few public hints that the debate had become more than just a 'professional' dispute among scientists; it had also taken on a personal animus (motivated perhaps by the differing political views of the disputants). When Greenwood made a passing reference to the 'illogical inferences' of 'X' on the subject of women and the vote, this constituted a not-very-veiled jab at Wright's public condemnation of female suffrage as 'militant hysteria' in a letter to the *Times*.[39] Even though the biometricians usually kept this 'private' aspect of the debate out of their public pronouncements, they actually saw Wright's attempt to use his standing as a medical researcher to make 'definitive' pronouncements on the political question of female suffrage as a further manifestation of the illogicality he had already demonstrated in discussing the opsonic index. As Pearson piquantly observed to Greenwood, 'It is curious when a man fails in logic in one matter, opsonic index, he is almost certain to fail in all things. Of course that does not in the least excuse his making a thorough cad of himself, or asking straight for sex war.'[40]

Despite this interesting personal aside, the main thrust of Greenwood's response to Wright's belief in individual expertise sounded some very Pearsonian intellectual notes. As an instance of the dangers of basing scientific conclusions on the 'consensus of expert opinion as a guide to truth' rather than an impersonal quantitative methodology, Greenwood cited the historical example of the widespread support that had once existed for the practice of bloodletting. In view of the fact that 'experts' have been in error in the past, Greenwood concluded that the 'rehabilitation of dogma and expert infallibility' must be abandoned and he explicitly reiterating Pearson's injunction that 'the day of authority in any branch of science *has* gone by'.[41]

Ultimately, the dispute between Wright and the biometricians over the merits of vaccine therapy and the opsonic index never reached definitive 'closure' (in the sense that both sides came to an agreement). Rather, each side went its separate way unconvinced of the validity of its adversary's point of view. As a case study of a scientific controversy, therefore, the debate terminated more as a result of what has been called 'natural death' or 'abandonment'[42] than by virtue of any definitive intellectual resolution of the issues at hand. However, this inability of the disputants to achieve consensus actually highlights fundamental disciplinary, philosophical, and political differences underscored by the disagreement.

At a disciplinary level, the dispute between Wright and the biometrical school reflects the long-standing dichotomy between the active experimental sciences (as exemplified by the laboratory) and the passive observational sciences (in this instance biometry). The contrast is nicely highlighted by the dispute over the relative merits of 'functional' and 'mathematical' error. For Wright, the active process of experimentally measuring the variations in the opsonic indices was more important in reaching a conclusion than any analyses of the opsonic index measurements performed (after the fact) by the biometricians; active experimentation could trump passive analysis. For the biometricians, by contrast, the essence of science consisted in the statistical analysis of quantitative data; the process of mathematical manipulation was more important than having an intimate knowledge of how that data were collected experimentally in the laboratory. The extent of the biometricians' loyalty to a vision of science that was primarily observational and mathematical is clearly illustrated by the fact that Pearson cited astronomy (the oldest of the mathematical non-experimental sciences[43]) as the prime example that 'functional error' could not supersede 'mathematical error' as Wright had maintained.

At a philosophical level, the debate over the existence of 'crucial experiments' illustrates fundamentally contrasting views about the nature of causality in science. Since the hallmark of a crucial experiment was that it generated 'always the same result' which could be interpreted as a 'universal truth', its existence was predicated ultimately on the ontological assumption that the natural world had a determinative causal structure. Thus, Wright's belief in crucial experiments reflects his implicit commitment to what (in contemporary philosophical parlance) would be called scientific realism, i.e., the view that correct scientific theories can be construed as true representations of the way that the world 'really' works even

141

if those theories postulated unobservable phenomena. For a thoroughgoing positivist (and anti-realist) such as Karl Pearson, by contrast, one was not permitted to posit the independent existence of unobservable attributes (such as causality) in describing the natural world; all a scientist could do was provide a clear description of what he or she observed empirically and measure the degree of association between these directly-observable antecedents and consequents. For this reason, correlation was seen as a much more fundamental organising construct for scientific inquiry than causality (which referred only to the limit case of unitary correlation). As Pearson observed in *The Grammar of Science*:

> The very statement of the law of causation involves antecedents – sameness of causes – which are purely conceptual and never actual. Permanence and absence of individuality in the bricks of the physical universe are only demonstrated in the same way that the bricks of a building are for many statistical purposes without individuality. The exact repetition of any antecedents is never possible, and all we can do is to classify things into like within a certain degree of observation, and record whether what we note as following from them are like within another degree of observation. Whenever we do this in physics, in zoology, in botany, in sociology, in medicine, or in any other branch of science, we really form a contingency table, and the causation of the physicist solely results from the fact not that the contingency coefficient of everything physical is unity but that he has so far worked to most profit in the field, where his contingency is so near unity that he could conceptualise his relationships as mathematical functions.[44]

Pearson's views had clearly influenced Greenwood who chose to respond to Wright's belief in crucial experiments by emphasising the human process by which scientific generalisations were formulated through multiple repetitions of experimental findings. Since no single experiment could conclusively establish any result, the emphasis was on how the individual scientist constructed theories about the world rather than on whether or not these theories 'corresponded' (in some relevant sense) to the way the world 'really' is; the focus was on science as method rather than subject matter.

Finally, the debate over the role of 'authoritative' opinion in science illustrates fundamentally different political visions as well as contrasting strategies of cultural legitimation for the scientific enterprise. By articulating a vision of science as a valid method for arriving at conclusions free from the biases of the individual mind,

Pearson proffered a vision of science that was a mirror image of his political views that put the concerns of society as a whole above those of the individual. Clearly recognising the political implications of Pearson's methodological statements, Wright rejected such a 'programme of socialistic egalitarianism' emphasising instead the 'exceptional skill' which the individual physician needed to make judgments in medicine. Thus, the feud between Wright and the biometricians actually played out in microcosm one of the perennial problematics that has bedevilled modern political theory of balancing the concerns of the individual with those of society at large.

Also, the debate over individual 'authority' versus statistical methods reflects contrasting rhetorical strategies of professional legitimation.[45] By emphasising a vision of science in which individual expertise was subordinated to universally-applicable quantitative methods, the biometricians articulated a fundamentally 'democratic' sense of professional legitimacy that provided no role for 'elites' with technical skills unique to their particular discipline[46]; as a result, the boundaries separating the various scientific subdisciplines were effectively eliminated. For Wright, by contrast, the existence of medicine as a clearly distinct intellectual pursuit was central to his sense of professional self-definition. In this regard, his invocation of the Hippocratic aphorism regarding the difficulty of medical judgment is especially telling; from antiquity to the present-day, the Hippocratic writings have been an important source for articulating the normative underpinnings for the view that medicine was a distinct science, which could be practised only by those suitably trained.

These differing visions of professional legitimacy are cast into especially bold relief when one contrasts the biometrical critique of Wright's work with the contemporary debate over vaccine therapy held before the Royal Society of Medicine in 1910. Even though the participating clinicians and bacteriologists disagreed profoundly about the relative merits of Wright's specific diagnostic and therapeutic claims, both sides actively embraced a conception of professional legitimacy based on an elite body of technical knowledge that one learned primarily through the concrete exigencies of disciplinary practice. For this reason, they portrayed the relationship between the clinician and the bacteriologist as symbiotic rather than adversarial.[47] As one commentator noted: 'If vaccine therapy is to take its right place as the handmaid to both medicine and surgery, every practitioner, whether specialist or general, must, of necessity, be expert in rudimentary bacteriological technique.'[48] Similarly, J. Kingston Fowler observed that 'as a student and subsequently he [the physician] must have received a careful and prolonged laboratory training. But I submit that he must continue to be in the future as he has been in the past, above all things a man of wide clinical experience.'[49] Arthur Latham made the point even more explicitly when he emphasised that 'we [the clinician and the bacteriologist] must work together, and … we must have at least a working knowledge of each other's subjects. There can be no rivalry between us. We have each of us a part, and an important part to play, and I trust that this discussion will do something to harmonise our respective fields of labour.'[50] Even though the clinician and the bacteriologist emphasised different types of expertise, their common focus on individually-acquired skill through experience shows the fundamental chasm separating both of them from the point of view of the biometrician who believed that the essence of science lay in an impersonal method for describing and analysing data.

In sum, even though the debate between Wright and the biometricians was ostensibly about highly technical diagnostic and therapeutic procedures (vaccine therapy and the opsonic index), the dichotomies presented by the two sides actually illustrate perennial questions about the nature of scientific inquiry as well as the interactive relationship of science to its larger social and cultural settings. By highlighting the multifaceted nature of such an interaction, debates such as this go along way toward challenging (what Andrew Pickering has called) 'the very frameworks and boundaries within which technical argument is conducted'.[51] As such, the dispute over the opsonic index proves to be significant not only because it was one of the first diagnostic tools that was subjected to biometric critique, but also because it illustrates what is arguably a defining feature within the contemporary historiography of science and medicine – the 'multidisciplinarity' inherent in scientific debate.

Notes

1. This paper is a further development of my earlier work originally published in the *Bulletin of the History of Medicine*, lxix (1995); and *Quantification and the Quest for Medical Certainty* (Princeton: Princeton University Press, 1995), ch. 5., 85–114.

2. See Leonard Colebrook, *Almroth Wright: Provocative Doctor and Thinker* (London: William Heinemann, 1954) 11–18; 'Wright, Sir Almroth Edward' in Richard R. Trail (ed.), *Munk's Roll* (London: Royal College of Physicians of London, 1968), 460–1; for an account of the typhoid debate, see Matthews *op. cit.* (note 1), 98–101.

3. Zachary Cope, *Almroth Wright: Founder of Modern Vaccine-Therapy*

(London: Thomas Nelson, 1966), 39–45.

4. Major Greenwood, 'A Statistical View of the Opsonic Index', *Proceedings of the Royal Society of Medicine*, ii, pt. 3 (1909), 146.

5. W. F. Harvey and Anderson McKendrick, 'The Opsonic Index – A Medico-Statistical Enquiry', *Biometrika*, vii (1909/1910), 65.

6. Almroth E. Wright, *Principles of Microscopy, being a handbook to the Microscope* (London: Archibald Constable & Co., Ltd, 1906), vi–vii.

7. Almroth E. Wright, 'Vaccine Therapy: Its Administration, Value, and Limitations. An Address Introductory to a Discussion on the Subject', *Proceedings of the Royal Society of Medicine*, iii, pt. 1 (1910), 29.

8. Almroth E. Wright to Major Greenwood, 18 November 1910, attached to letter from Greenwood to Karl Pearson, 20 November 1910, box 707, Karl Pearson Papers. I would like to thank the Library University College London for permission to quote from the Karl Pearson Papers, subsequently cited as KPP. Also, I would like to thank Cina Wong, C. D. E., for assistance in deciphering Wright's nearly illegible handwriting.

9. Karl Pearson, *The Grammar of Science*, 3rd edn (New York: Macmillan, 1911), 6.

10. See, *ibid.*, 55.

11. Theodore M. Porter, 'The Death of the Object: *Fin de siècle* Philosophy of Physics', in Dorothy Ross (ed.), *Modernist Impulses in the Human Sciences, 1870-1930* (Baltimore: Johns Hopkins University Press, 1994), 143–50.

12. Wright, *op. cit.* (note 7), 28.

13. Karl Pearson, 'The Opsonic Index – 'Mathematical Error and Functional Error" *Biometrika* viii (1911–12), 203–4.

14. *Ibid.*, 204.

15. *Ibid.*, 210.

16. *Ibid.*, 211.

17. *Ibid.*, 221.

18. Almroth E. Wright, *Handbook of the Technique of the Teat and Capillary Glass Tube, And its Applications in Medicine and Bacteriology* (London: Constable & Company, Ltd, 1912), 163.

19. See, *ibid.*, 164–5.

20. On the place of Wright and the broader efforts at producing pneumococcal vaccines in the first half of the twentieth century, see Peter C. English, 'Therapeutic Strategies to Combat Pneumococcal Disease: Repeated Failure of Physicians to Adopt Pneumococcal Vaccine', *Perspectives in Biology and Medicine*, xxx (1987), 170–185, esp. 173–5.

21. Almroth E. Wright *et al.*, 'Observations on the Pharmaco-Therapy

of Pneumococcus Infections', *The Lancet* (December 14, 1912), 1636.

22. See *ibid.*, 1636.
23. Almroth E. Wright *et al.*, 'Observations on the Pharmaco-Therapy of Pneumococcus Infections', *Lancet* (December 21, 1912), 1701.
24. See *ibid.*, 1702.
25. See *ibid.*, 1702.
26. See *ibid.*, 1702.
27. See *ibid.*, 1703.
28. Pearson to Greenwood, 17 December 1912, box 915, KPP.
29. See *ibid.*
30. See Greenwood's autobiographical statement (1924) in Greenwood file, Raymond Pearl Papers, American Philosophical Society, Philadelphia, 1-8; Lancelot Hogben, 'Major Greenwood, 1880-1949', *Obituary Notices of Fellows of the Royal Society*, vii (1950-51), 141.
31. C. J. Martin to Major Greenwood, 18 November 1909, and Greenwood to Martin, 20 November 1909, 'Miscellaneous correspondence re appointments, 1909-25', Lister Institute Archives in the Contemporary Medical Archives Centre at the Wellcome Institute for the History of Medicine, 183 Euston Road, London NW1 2BP, CMAC: SA/LIS/H.9.
32. Major Greenwood to Karl Pearson, 24 June 1909, box 707, KPP.
33. Major Greenwood, 'On Methods of Research Available in the Study of Medical Problems, With Special Reference to Sir Almroth Wright's Recent Utterances', *Lancet* (January 18, 1913), 160.
34. See *ibid.*, 163.
35. See *ibid.*, 160–1.
36. This distinction eerily presages by a quarter of a century the famous distinction that Hans Reichenbach would make between the 'context of discovery' and the 'context of justification', cf. *Experience and Prediction: An Analysis of the Foundations and the Structure of Knowledge* (Chicago: University of Chicago Press, 1938), 6–7.
37. Greenwood, *op. cit.* (note 33), 162.
38. See *ibid.*; Pearson, *op. cit.* (note 9), 55.
39. 'Sir Almroth Wright on Militant Hysteria', *The Times* (28 March 1912), 7-8.
40. Pearson to Greenwood, 29 March 1912, box 915, KPP.
41. Greenwood, *op. cit.* (note 33), 164.
42. See Tom L. Beauchamp, 'Ethical theory and the problem of closure', in H. Tristram Englehardt, Jr. and Arthur Caplan (eds), *Scientific Controversies: Case Studies in the Resolution and Closure of Dispute in Science and Technology* (Cambridge: Cambridge University Press,

1987), 27–48; and Ernan McMullin, 'Scientific controversy and its termination', in H. Tristram Englehardt, Jr. and Arthur Caplan (eds), *Scientific Controversies: Case Studies in the Resolution and Closure of Dispute in Science and Technology* (Cambridge: Cambridge University Press, 1987), 49–91

43. On astronomy as the oldest non-experimental science, see Thomas S. Kuhn's famous article, 'Mathematical versus Experimental Traditions in the Development of Physical Science', in *idem, The Essential Tension: Selected Studies in Scientific Tradition and Change* (Chicago: University of Chicago Press, 1977), 31–65.

44. Pearson, *op. cit.* (note 9), 164-5.

45. On the role of rhetoric in methodological debates about science and medicine in this period, see Richard R.Yeo, 'Scientific Method and the Rhetoric of Science in Britain, 1830-1914', in John A. Schuster and Richard R. Yeo (eds), *The Politics and Rhetoric of Science Method* (Dordrecht: Reidel Publishing Company, 1986), 259–97; and Christopher Lawrence, 'Incommunicable Knowledge: Science, Technology, and the Clinical Art in Britain, 1850–1914' *Journal of Contemporary History,* xx (1985), 503–20.

46. On the role of quantification and modern democratic political institutions more generally, see Theodore M. Porter, *Trust in Numbers: The Pursuit of Objectivity in Science and Public Life* (Princeton: Princeton University Press, 1995).

47. This point is made very cogently in an American context in Russell C. Maulitz, "Physician Versus Bacteriologist': The Ideology of Science in Clinical Medicine', in Morris J. Vogel and Charles E. Rosenberg (eds), *The Therapeutic Revolution: Essays in the Social History of American Medicine* (Philadelphia: University of Pennsylvania Press, 1979), 91–107.

48. A. Butler Harris, *Proceedings of the Royal Society of Medicine,* iii, pt. 1 (1910), 102.

49. J. Kingston Fowler, in *ibid.,* 110.

50. Arthur Latham, in *ibid.,* 128.

51. Andrew Pickering, 'From Science as Knowledge to Science as Practice', in Andrew Pickering (ed.), *Science as Practice and Culture* (Chicago: University of Chicago Press, 1992), 7.

Index